Fertility Facts

Fertility Facts

Hundreds of Tips for Getting Pregnant

By Kim Hahn
and the Editors of
Conceive Magazine

Foreword by
Jennifer L. Howse, Ph.D., President, March of Dimes

CHRONICLE BOOKS
SAN FRANCISCO

Library of Congress Cataloging-in-Publication Data available.

ISBN: 978-0-8118-6421-3

Manufactured in China

Design by Patrick Greenish
Indexed by Michelle Graye

Based on articles written for Conceive Magazine: Founder, Kim Hahn; Editor-in-Chief, Beth Weinhouse; Managing Editor, Stephanie Pancratz; Art Director, Patrick Greenish.

10 9 8 7 6 5 4 3 2 1

Chronicle Books LLC
680 Second Street
San Francisco, California 94107
www.chroniclebooks.com

www.conceiveonline.com

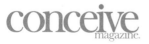

❧ Contents ❧

Foreword

For many couples, getting pregnant is easy. For many others, it takes a bit longer than expected. And for some, it may even require medical help. For all of these people—in other words, for anyone hoping to become a parent of a healthy baby—knowledge can be the key to success. Knowing how your reproductive system works, why preconception health is so important, and what changes you can make in your lifestyle to increase your fertility will help couples at any stage of the journey. Small changes can sometimes make the difference between success and another month of trying.

At the March of Dimes, our mission is to help women have healthy babies, and we believe that one of the most important steps toward that goal is preparation, which includes education about fertility and pregnancy. That's where *Conceive Magazine* and its new publication, *Fertility Facts,* come in. It's never too early—or too late—to learn more about the process of conception and pregnancy. In this new book, *Conceive* shares easy-to-understand information about many of the issues that can potentially affect fertility, for better or worse.

It's also a good idea to develop a reproductive life plan, which simply means that couples should discuss ahead of time if and when they want to get pregnant. The March of Dimes finds that having a timetable helps women and their partners get as healthy as possible before pregnancy—whether that means quitting smoking, losing weight, or any other lifestyle or health change—in order to have healthier pregnancies and babies. To create such a plan, make an appointment with a health care provider. *Fertility Facts* provides valuable information about the preconception checkup and what should be discussed. You can also find more information at www.marchofdimes.com and www.nacersano.org (our Spanish-language site), including important issues to consider concerning fertility treatments.

Learn the facts about fertility before you begin trying to get pregnant, and then continue educating yourself once you've conceived. *Fertility Facts* and the March of Dimes will provide you with all the information you need to sort through the latest medical and scientific research, and take charge of your healthy lifestyle. Those are the best things you can do to achieve pregnancy and give your baby a full and healthy nine-month start to life.

Jennifer L. Howse, Ph.D.
President
March of Dimes

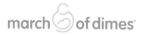

The Preconception Checkup

The March of Dimes recommends that women ask their health care providers the following questions at a preconception checkup, and discuss these issues before trying to get pregnant.

- Do I have any ongoing health conditions such as diabetes, high blood pressure, lupus, or heart disease that need to be better controlled before pregnancy?
- Are my vaccinations and immunizations for infections like chickenpox, measles, mumps, and rubella up to date? Do I have any current infections that need treatment?
- Am I at increased risk because someone in my family had a baby born before 37 weeks?
- Will any of the medications I'm taking hinder conception or pose a pregnancy risk?
- Do I have any bad habits, such as smoking or excessive drinking, that may pose a risk to pregnancy, and how can I get help to quit?
- How can I reduce the stress in my life, or learn to handle it better?
- How can I improve my diet and nutrition?
- Should I begin taking a multivitamin containing 400 micrograms of folic acid every day, or even a prenatal vitamin?

Introduction

Everyone knows how babies are made, right? The truth is, most people just know the basics. Way beyond the birds-and-bees talk from parents, and far further even than high school sex ed, is a world of information about human reproduction and how it works, why it sometimes doesn't, and what can help.

In fact, fertility is something most people take for granted until they decide it's time to start a family. And then, suddenly, all the lifestyle decisions made earlier in life become relevant in a new way. Diet, exercise, sexual practices, and medical history all play a part in determining whether the journey to parenthood will be a straight path or a route with many detours.

Reproductive health is often a reflection of general health. But, as with so many health issues, it's just not that simple. After all, it takes two to make a baby. So one member of a couple may be in tip-top reproductive shape, but if the other isn't, there can still be challenges conceiving. Sometimes minor health problems that would have remained hidden forever, because they have no symptoms, become a factor. And sometimes it's impossible to determine why it's so easy for some people to get pregnant, and more of a long-term project for others.

The 250 facts in this book are not exactly secrets, but they're not widely known, either. For instance, did you know that cell phones may affect fertility? Soybeans? That women who drink whole milk rather than skim have a reproductive advantage? That biological clocks don't just tick the years, but the seasons, too? These are just a few examples of the hundreds

Introduction

of fascinating facts that fill this book. The information is drawn from a wide variety of sources, including scientific journals, government statistics, medical experts, and alternative practitioners.

The book is divided into ten chapters, each with its own theme. All of the chapters include a mix of important, fun, serious, and interesting facts. The first nine chapters deal with basic reproductive function, diet and exercise, vitamins and supplements, and other information that ranges from basic to esoteric, but probably wasn't taught in high school health class. And almost all of the facts include a recommendation that can help couples use the information to maximize their fertility and get pregnant faster. Armed with this knowledge, couples will know everything they need to know to speed up their own journey . . . and they'll also know how to recognize when it's time to get help from an OB-GYN or reproductive endocrinologist.

Since 2004, *Conceive Magazine* has been keeping tabs on every aspect of fertility to help couples achieve their dreams of starting or expanding their families. The magazine's reporters have tracked down the biggest medical experts and interviewed nurses, doctors, scientific researchers, psychologists and life coaches, practitioners of Traditional Chinese Medicine, egg and sperm donors (and recipients), and more. *Conceive's* writers have sifted through medical journals, analyzed data from many sources, and sometimes challenged prevailing wisdom. All to present readers with the most up-to-date and accurate information possible. Much of that information is now collected here, and presented as easily digested, logically organized, bite-size bits of information that all together provide a sumptuous meal of reproductive knowledge.

Read through from beginning to end if you like, but it's certainly not necessary to consume these 250 facts in order. Check out Chapter 2 if you want a crash course in how your monthly cycle works. Skip to Chapter 8 on men's health if you're concerned about your partner's fertility. Peek at Chapter 9, about sex, before you head to the bedroom tonight. (Do you think you need to lie in bed with your legs in the air after sex to maximize your chance of conceiving? Turn to page 230: you might be surprised!)

These facts pack volumes of information in easily digestible bits that will make you feel informed, but not overwhelmed. As you read, remember the vast majority of couples who want to start a family will be pregnant within the year. For those who aren't, medical science now offers an arsenal of treatments, both high- and low-tech, to help. The subject of Chapter 10, the final chapter, is assisted reproduction and other fertility treatments. For couples who are concerned that their journey is taking longer than they expected, this chapter provides explanations of what may be happening to prevent pregnancy, and what can be done to overcome the obstacle.

And when you're ready to start trying, you can use this information and chart your journey in *Conceive Magazine's The Fertility Journal: A Day-by-Day Guide to Getting Pregnant* (Chronicle Books, 2008). This book not only contains important information about fertility and conception, but also tips for dealing with the up-and-down emotions of the fertility roller coaster, and what to expect once you get that positive pregnancy test. Plus plenty of space to chart your own information—doctors appointments, cycle dates, vitamins and medications—along the way.

Whether you're thinking about "trying" next year, planning to start in a few months, or you're already working on your baby project, the following information can help prepare you for the quickest possible conception, and the healthiest possible pregnancy. Good luck on your journey.

Chapter
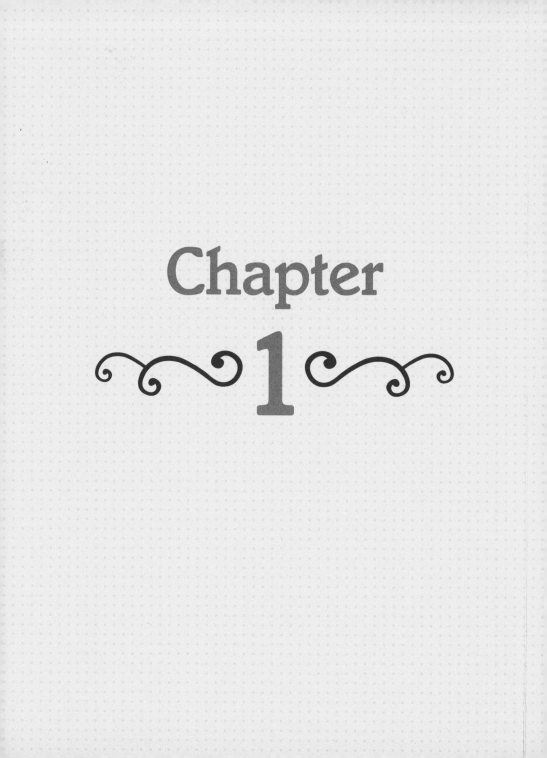

1

Before You Conceive

If you've been thinking of pregnancy as a nine-month project, remember to factor in some prep time. There's lots to be done before you conceive to make sure your body is in the best shape possible to not only conceive a child, but also to carry a healthy pregnancy to term. In other words, you've got to take care of your own health before you can take care of your baby's. Before you start "trying" is the time to take stock of your own health and lifestyle, and see what needs changing. Here are some recommendations for things to do, check, and get under control before the babymaking project begins.

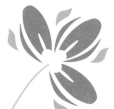

Visit Your Doctor

Scheduling a preconception checkup before you even try to get pregnant is one of the best steps you can take to ensure a healthy path for you and your baby-to-be. It's even part of the latest advice from the Centers for Disease Control and Prevention (CDC). Talking to a doctor about any lifestyle issues that might affect babymaking makes sense for every woman, but is especially important for women with chronic health conditions such as diabetes, high blood pressure, mood disorders, or epilepsy. A preconception checkup can help you get a handle on what pregnancy will mean for you and the best ways to handle your health while you're gestating.

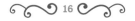

Make Sure Your Partner Gets a Checkup, Too

Many women may know it's important to schedule a preconception appointment before they try to become pregnant, but you may not realize it's equally important for your partner to have a checkup as well. Male fertility can be negatively affected by a variety of lifestyle choices, including smoking, exposure to environmental hazards, recreational drug use, or even just extreme stress. Because sperm develop over a three-month period, men should try to eliminate any negative impacts for at least those three months before trying to conceive.

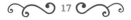

Honesty Is the Most Fertile Policy

When you're trying to conceive, it's important to be completely honest with your doctor. And that means about everything. Physicians need to have a complete picture of what's going on with your and your partner's bodies, even if that means "fessing up" to recreational drug use, smoking, excessive drinking, and any sexually transmitted diseases you may have had in the past. Previous abortions or miscarriages can also affect present fertility. If you're hiding something like this in your past from your partner, know the doctor will ask about it. Honesty with your partner is the best policy, of course. If need be, ask for a private consult with your physician to explain your history and concerns.

A Shot of Prevention

At your preconception checkup, make sure to go over your vaccination history with your doctor. It's especially important that pregnant women have up-to-date chicken pox (varicella) and rubella (German measles) protection, since these diseases can cause problems during the first or third trimester of pregnancy. Because both these shots are live vaccines—meaning they include all or part of a usually weakened disease-causing organism—they're not recommended during pregnancy. Some routine shots, such as the tetanus/diphtheria shot that adults are advised to have every ten years, are considered safe during pregnancy, but it's still smartest to get vaccinations up-to-date before you conceive.

Get Your Periods on Track

It's no secret that a regular menstrual cycle is a sign of fertility and an irregular cycle could signal problems. Stress, depression, and being under- or overweight all can affect a woman's menstrual cycle. If none of these obvious causes seem to be a factor for you, consult a physician. Skipped or irregular periods could signal an underlying medical problem, like polycystic ovary syndrome (PCOS), or some other hormonal imbalance. For otherwise healthy women who simply have irregular cycles, doctors recommend trying ovulation predictor kits to zero in on the most fertile time of the cycle.

Look into Your Family Tree

No one can guarantee a healthy baby, but getting genetic testing before you conceive can help you and your partner spot some potential problems before you become pregnant. Your family history and your family background will determine which tests might be recommended. For instance, African-Americans should be tested for sickle cell anemia. Individuals of Ashkenazi Jewish descent are at increased risk of several genetic disorders, including Tay-Sachs, Canavan, Gaucher, and familial dysautonomia. People of Southeast Asian and Mediterranean ancestry should be screened for alpha and beta thalassemias. And all couples should consider testing for cystic fibrosis. A genetic test will determine if one or both parents carry the specific genetic mutation, and what the risk is of passing that mutation on to a child. Often, potential parents will not have symptoms themselves, but if both partners are carriers, children can be affected. Schedule a consultation with a genetic counselor or doctor who can advise you about evaluating individual risks and deciding on the best course of action.

Before You Conceive

Take Care of Your Mental Health

If you think you only need to take care of yourself from the neck down to get ready for Baby, think again. The brain is the real "fertility boss" because it regulates the hormones that affect the reproductive organs. Struggling with stress or depression while trying to conceive can throw up roadblocks in the reproductive pathway. If you're having trouble handling something in your life, talk to a mental health professional to find the best path of relief for your situation.

Fertility Facts

Pre-Prenatal Vitamins

You undoubtedly know about prenatal vitamins—those usually large supplements that are handed out to pregnant women at their first prenatal checkup. But now many doctors are advising women who know they want to be pregnant soon to start taking the vitamins even before they conceive. Regular one-a-day type vitamins, which contain at least 400 micrograms of folic acid will work fine, or you can opt for one of the prenatal vitamin formulas that are now sold over-the-counter (without a prescription). Folic acid is especially important, since it helps prevent some devastating birth defects that can occur very early in pregnancy, before many women even realize they've conceived.

Investigate Your Medicine Cabinet

Most women know they have to worry about what medicines are safe when they're pregnant, but few mommies-in-the-making realize that drugs taken while trying to conceive can affect fertility. A few examples of common pills that can subtly sabotage reproduction include antidepressants (which can increase levels of the hormone prolactin, possibly blocking ovulation); antihistamines (some of which may inhibit implantation of an egg into the womb); and decongestants (which can not only dry up a runny nose, but potentially dry out the mucous membranes responsible for creating a friendly environment for sperm to travel into the uterus and fallopian tubes to fertilize an egg). Long-term use of corticosteroids and some pain relievers can also have an impact. It's best to talk to your doctor about any medications you take, including over-the-counter and herbal formulas, before trying to conceive.

Get Chronic Health Conditions Under Control

Taking care of your body is the best way to prepare for Baby, and that means getting chronic conditions under control, especially when they can affect fertility. For example, thyroid conditions are important to screen for and treat early on, since they can not only affect fertility, but also can be tricky to treat during gestation. Doctors suggest that women who have diabetes get their blood glucose levels under control three to six months before they become pregnant, and continue close monitoring during pregnancy. It's smart to ask your doctor about any health issue that you deal with to find out how it might affect conception and pregnancy.

Before You Conceive

Two to Avoid

Two medications are considered so dangerous during pregnancy that doctors advise women to stop taking them (and switch to a safer drug if necessary) even before they're pregnant. These drugs are the blood thinner warfarin (brand name Coumadin) and isotretinoins used to treat acne (Accutane, Amnesteem, Claravis, and Sotret). Women who take these drugs but who want to get pregnant are strongly advised to switch, since the medications are known to cause birth defects, infant death, miscarriage, and premature delivery. By stopping or switching before you conceive, you eliminate the risk of exposing your baby in the earliest weeks of pregnancy, before you realize you're pregnant.

Count Your Eggs Before You Conceive

Women 35 and older are often acutely aware that their "egg supply" is on the decline. While a literal "egg count" is impossible, the most accurate test for what is medically called "ovarian reserve" involves measuring the blood level of follicle stimulating hormone (FSH). FSH is produced by the pituitary gland and helps direct the ovaries to mature and release eggs. A rising FSH level indicates a decreasing egg supply, as the pituitary gland pumps out more of the hormone to stimulate ovaries that are no longer responding as they once did. Because the timing of the test is important, women will get the most accurate results by consulting their doctor rather than relying on an over-the-counter test.

Before You Conceive

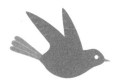

Remember to Floss

A gynecologist isn't the only health expert you'll want to visit before pregnancy; a dentist may also have a hand in helping a woman have a healthy pregnancy. Gum disease, such as gingivitis (inflammation of the gums) and periodontitis (more advanced gum disease), has been associated with the risk of preterm delivery and low-birthweight babies, so schedule a preconception dental cleaning and exam. Your home hygiene (brushing and flossing) is very important, but if you need to have any dental work that involves X-rays or medications, you're best off taking care of these things before you conceive.

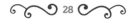

Time to Smile

If you've been thinking about brightening your smile, act fast. Right now, doctors don't know for sure whether the bleaches used to whiten teeth are safe during pregnancy, so they generally advise pregnant women to wait until after delivery before making their pearly whites even whiter. But if you don't want to wait that long, it's best to lighten up now. Just think, soon you'll have lots to smile about!

You Can Turn Around a Tubal Ligation

More than 700,000 women in the United States undergo tubal ligations each year, and about 1 percent of those who choose to tie their tubes will eventually seek a reversal. While in vitro fertilization can get around this problem (by retrieving eggs directly from the ovaries and then implanting them in the uterus—in effect creating a detour around the fallopian tubes), many women prefer to have their surgeries reversed and try for babies the old-fashioned way. The procedure, called tubal anastomosis or tubal reanastomosis, is successful for many women who have had traditional tubal ligations and is an outpatient procedure with full recovery taking about two weeks. Women who have had the method of surgical sterilization called Essure®, however, should consider their sterilization permanent.

Conception and Contraception

The contraceptive you used before trying to become pregnant can make a difference in how long it will take you to conceive. There's good news for couples who relied on such barrier methods as condoms, diaphragms, and the cervical cap. The return to fertility is as simple as leaving them in your night table drawer. That's because barrier methods only work when they are on—or in—the body. Of course, they also help preserve your fertility by reducing your risk of sexually transmitted diseases, including chlamydia and gonorrhea, which can damage the reproductive organs. (For information on hormonal methods of contraception, and how to prepare for pregnancy if you've been using them, see the next page.)

Pick a Date to Go Off the Pill

Most women begin ovulating immediately after stopping hormonal birth control methods like the Pill. Ovulation should begin within weeks, says Paul Blumenthal, M.D., M.P.H., professor of obstetrics and gynecology at Stanford University School of Medicine in California. For some, however, it can take a few months to get menstrual cycles back on track. If you've been taking birth control pills and are planning to be pregnant soon, it's a good idea to pick the date you intend to start "trying," and then go off your oral contraceptives a few months before that date. Use a barrier method like condoms or a diaphragm for birth control until you're ready to start trying.

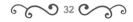

But Start Right Away if You'd Like

Doctors stress that women don't need to get the Pill "out of their systems" first for fear of harming their unborn child; many babies have been conceived while women were on the Pill, and they've shown no increased risk for birth defects. Most recent studies show that 80 percent of women who want to get pregnant will within a year after going off the Pill. One reason doctors sometimes advise women to wait a few months is that it will be easier to predict the due date of a pregnancy if a woman has had at least one normal, non-Pill menstrual cycle first. But if a woman does get pregnant after stopping the Pill but before having her period, a doctor can pinpoint the baby's due date through ultrasound.

The Pill Can Actually Promote Pregnancy

Not only is the Pill not linked with infertility, it may actually help preserve your babymaking ability by lowering your risk of uterine and ovarian cancers. If you've got endometriosis, in which the uterine lining grows outside the uterus, the Pill can suppress symptoms, potentially reducing the extent of scar tissue formation. In women with PCOS, it thins the outer coating that builds up on the ovary, reducing the production of abnormal hormones, says David B. Morehead, D.O., an OB-GYN at Baylor Medical Center at Waxahachie in Texas. But can the Pill help you get pregnant by regulating your cycle, as some women believe? Unlikely. That cycle regulation is artificial, say doctors. Once women go off the Pill, their fertility returns to whatever level it would have been. However, some women's cycles regulate themselves over time, regardless of whether or not they take the Pill.

Home, Safe Home

When most people think about environmental threats, they think about air and water pollution, or on-the-job exposures to hazardous chemicals. But don't forget that your environment includes your home; in fact, you probably spend more time there than anywhere else. So when you're trying to get pregnant, don't neglect to ensure that the house you live in is safe, too. To minimize exposure to possibly hazardous chemicals, consider switching to "green" cleaning products, "natural" cosmetics, and non-plastic food storage containers and utensils.

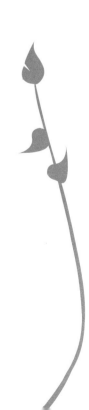

Know What's What on the Job

If you work in an environment where you're exposed to chemicals, make sure you know exactly what the chemicals are and what effect they may have on a pregnancy. Employers are required by law to release the Material Safety Data Sheets (MSDS) on any workplace chemicals to employees. If you're concerned about workplace chemical hazards, speak to your employer about changes you can make once you're pregnant (if not before). It's also important that your partner check his job exposures, as well; some chemicals can affect male fertility, too.

Fertility Facts

It May Take Time

While numerous studies have confirmed that hormonal birth control methods like Depo-Provera, intrauterine devices (IUDs), and patches do not cause infertility, it will take your body a few months to readjust to normal cycles after discontinuing one of these methods. It takes an average of ten months to conceive after your last contraceptive shot and twelve months or more after having an IUD removed.

Depo-Provera, a hormonal shot injected into women's arms or buttocks every three months, prevents pregnancy by halting ovulation and is not a good choice for women who hope to become pregnant right away. After the last shot, the median time for return to fertility is ten months, according to research. So far, there isn't long-term data on the Patch, which delivers a low dose of estrogen through the skin, or the Ring, which releases hormones for three weeks after being inserted in the vagina. As for the IUD, the return to fertility after removal is fairly rapid, somewhere between the rate of the Pill and Depo-Provera.

Before You Conceive

Fertile Women Come in All Sizes

Women of all shapes and sizes are able to get pregnant, so don't sweat what you can't change, doctors say. So-called childbearing hips might sometimes help with delivery, but they have nothing to do with fertility and conception. And while a 2004 study in the journal *Fertility and Sterility* did show that women with larger breasts and smaller waists have higher levels of the fertility-associated hormones estrogen and progesterone, the study didn't compare pregnancy rates. After all, women with flat chests and narrow hips get pregnant all the time. So rather than focusing on things you can't change, realize that you can conceive, no matter what your body shape. Instead of worrying about your measurements, concentrate on staying healthy and having sexual intercourse during your most fertile period.

Exercise Is Not a Fertility Drug

If you're in great shape and general good health, you've definitely got a fertility advantage. But don't make the mistake of assuming that your great BMI (body mass index), strong biceps, and fast running times means you've got nothing to worry about. Pat yourself on the back for taking such great care of your body, but don't neglect the preconception advice recommended for all women who are hoping to be pregnant soon. Fitness level is just one element of fertility. According to the American Pregnancy Association, couples who are actively trying to conceive have about a one-in-four chance in any given month. And that goes for both marathoners and couch potatoes.

Learn Your Mother's Fertility History

The older your mother was when you were conceived, the more likely you may be to have a fertility problem. That's the result of a study of 74 in vitro fertilization patients in Atlanta, Georgia, conducted by Zsolt Nagy, M.D. The study found that the women who weren't able to get pregnant had been conceived an average of twenty years before their mothers entered menopause, as opposed to an average of more than twenty-five years pre-menopause for the women who did achieve pregnancy. Dr. Nagy theorizes that genetic abnormalities from a mother's older eggs may have been passed down to the daughters. Obviously many factors go into the decision about when it's time to start a family, but if your mother had you later in life, you might want to add that information to the mix and consider putting your family plans on the fast track (or at least talk to your physician about your age and your fertility prospects).

Fertility Facts

Know When Your Mother's Periods Stopped

If you're trying to conceive after you're 40 years old, it's important to know when your mother entered menopause. If her periods stopped when she was in her late forties, you might consider putting your pregnancy on a fast track. While women are often advised to try for a year before consulting a fertility specialist, older women may want to be more proactive. If you're trying and haven't conceived in three to six months, consider consulting with a fertility specialist.

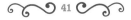

Chapter 2

Fertility Basics

Most of us probably think we understand basic human biology, including how our monthly cycles work, and—of course!—how babies are made. But the workings of the female reproductive system are so fascinating and so complex that biologists are still studying its mysteries and making new discoveries. The clockwork interaction of hormones that regulate ovulation are a sort of medical miracle. And the more you know about your own cycle—and specifically how to determine when you ovulate (release a ripened egg with the potential to be fertilized)—the better your chances of conceiving each month. Read on for a crash course in the female reproductive system.

You're Most Fertile BEFORE You Ovulate

Doctors used to tell couples to have intercourse before, during, or right after ovulation (when a ripened egg is released from the ovary), but they now know that women are most likely to get pregnant if they have sex in the 5 days before—or on the day of—ovulation, not after. That's because once an egg is released from the ovary, it's receptive to sperm for only 12 to 24 hours. Sperm, meanwhile, can remain viable for days—and sometimes weeks—after intercourse. So the more sperm present prior to ovulation, the better your chances of conception. Even women with perfect 28-day cycles, however, can ovulate irregularly. For this reason, most OB-GYNs recommend that couples trying to conceive have sex every other day for at least several weeks midcycle, to maximize the chances of sperm being present when an egg is released.

Fertility Facts

Count Backward to Pinpoint Ovulation

The biggest mistake women make when trying to become pregnant is miscalculating when they're ovulating. Many of us assume we ovulate on day 14 of our cycles, but this is only the case for women with regular 28-day cycles. What's more, ovulation doesn't occur 14 days *after* the start of menstruation, but 14 days *before*. The best way to determine when you're likely to ovulate: select the date you expect your next period to begin and subtract 14 days. Using this formula, a woman with a 24-day cycle will usually ovulate on day 10, while someone with a 30-day cycle can expect ovulation to occur on day 16. Interestingly, women may not be the best judges of their own cycles. An October 2007 study in the *American Journal of Epidemiology* found that, on average, women overestimated their cycle lengths by nearly a day.

Sugar and Spice . . . and Lots of Eggs

A baby girl is born with all her eggs—1 to 2 million—already inside her ovaries. Men can usually produce sperm their entire lives, but for women it's all a numbers game. Every month for about twenty-five years, our ovaries release a single mature egg, for a total of 300 during our reproductive years. Yet at birth our ovaries contain more than 1 million eggs, all our bodies will ever produce. The first day of our lives, immature eggs begin to self-destruct and are absorbed by the body, a process known as atresia. By puberty, a girl has about 300,000 eggs remaining. Our eggs are at their peak during our mid-to-late twenties. By our thirties, we may have plenty of eggs left, but the follicles that surround and release them become less responsive to hormonal signals. Why some women exhaust their egg supply at a young age, while others have no trouble getting pregnant and delivering healthy babies in their late thirties and forties is unknown. We each have a unique biological clock that's set to a very individualized timer.

Fertility Facts

The Average Age of Menopause in the United States Is Fifty

Your mother's—and even your grandmother's—age at menopause may give you a clue to your own. Women in the developed world reach this last reproductive milestone at around 50 years, on average. (For a variety of genetic and environmental factors, in rural, developing countries the average age of menopause is earlier: around age 43.) If your mother or grandmother had an early menopause, you're apt to follow suit. Likewise, if they didn't stop menstruating until their early to mid-fifties, you may gain a longer stretch of fertile years. But this isn't cast in stone. A special workshop on Stages of Reproductive Aging, hosted by the National Institutes of Health in 2001, noted that individual women may be born with "a highly variable number of oocytes [eggs]" and that the rate at which they lose eggs also varies greatly. So talk to Mom, but remember, biology isn't necessarily destiny.

Fertility Basics

Reproductive Aging Begins Earlier Than You Think

From a biological perspective, the peak ages for a woman to have a baby are between 18 and 20. Women's fertility actually starts to decline in the late twenties, men's after age 35, according to a 2002 study in *Human Reproduction*. Researchers from the United States and Italy studied 782 healthy couples and estimated the chances of pregnancy following intercourse two days prior to ovulation, the peak time for conception. Women ages 19 to 26 whose partner was the same age had about a 50 percent chance of pregnancy in any one menstrual cycle. This fell to 40 percent for women 27 to 34, and less than 30 percent for women 35 to 39, unless their partner was 5 years older, at which point the pregnancy rate dropped to 20 percent. The good news: this did not mean a lower overall chance of achieving pregnancy if women delayed trying until their late twenties or early thirties, the researchers noted. It meant that it may take women in their late twenties a month or two longer to become pregnant than it would have earlier in that decade.

Fertility Facts

The Forties Can Still Be Fertile

It's almost a mantra: after age 40 a woman isn't likely to conceive using her own eggs because her cycles are so irregular. Yet about two-thirds of women between the ages of 40 and 44 continue to ovulate regularly. To determine how much life is left in your eggs, you can get a simple blood test that measures the level of follicle stimulating hormone (FSH). Produced by the pituitary gland, it helps control the menstrual cycle and the production of eggs. In another test, called the clomiphene challenge test, your doctor prescribes a course of five days of clomiphene citrate and then measures your FSH level afterward. The idea is to stimulate the ovaries and see how quickly they respond, an indication of your ovarian reserves. If you're in your forties and your doctor doesn't offer these tests, insist on them. If you're not producing quality eggs, the sooner you know the quicker you can chart a plan of action.

Fertility Basics

40-Year-Old Eggs May Not Be Grade A

The majority of women still ovulate into their forties, but they're less likely to produce high-quality eggs. A major reason is "There can be metabolic changes in the eggs," that reduce their quality, says Lynn Westphal, MD, associate professor of obstetrics and gynecology at the Stanford University School of Medicine in California. What's more, "it's well documented that at age 40, half of the eggs a woman produces are chromosomally abnormal," she says. As a result, while women may still conceive in their forties, they're more likely to suffer early miscarriages.

Fertility Facts

Luck Be a Baby Tonight

Everyone knows some enviable couples who conceive the first month they try. But paying undue attention to the quick conceivers in your life can set up unrealistic expectations for you. Women who aren't pregnant within the first few months, for instance, may be convinced they're infertile when they're not. The truth is that couples have approximately a 15 percent chance of conceiving each month they have unprotected intercourse—and it takes an average of eight months for them to get pregnant.

Fertility Basics

The Twenties: Fast Track to Parenthood

When it comes to conception, chronological age can make a difference. Women are most fertile in their twenties, when they have a 25 percent chance of conceiving each month. That's because by then, they're usually having regular cycles and producing robust eggs, which ripen and are released by the ovaries on schedule each month. Not surprisingly, "there aren't many women in their twenties who have infertility," says Lynn Westphal, MD, associate professor of obstetrics and gynecology at the Stanford University School of Medicine in California. Although these are peak years for egg maturation and release, be aware that it still takes an average of four to five months to conceive, and six to seven if you're in your late twenties.

Thirty-something Conception

About 20 percent of women put off childbearing until after age 35, according to the American Society of Reproductive Medicine (ASRM). Not only are more women working today, but they're marrying at an older age. And some couples prefer to wait until they're more financially secure before bringing a baby on board. Delaying pregnancy until this decade won't necessarily wreak reproductive havoc, despite the doom-and-gloom attitude of some reproductive endocrinologists. The good news: when a woman reaches her thirties, she usually still has a plentiful supply of eggs. The bad: beginning around the middle of the decade, egg quality becomes less reliable. This explains why women in their thirties have a reduced 10 to 15 percent chance of conceiving each month, and it will take an average of seven to twelve months to conceive.

Beating the Odds in the Forties

As women age, so do the eggs in their ovaries. And when these older eggs are fertilized, they're less likely than younger ones to develop. If you're in your forties, your chance of conceiving is 5 percent each month, dropping precipitously as you approach 50. The ovaries may be responding poorly to follicle stimulating hormone (FSH), which stimulates the production of eggs, and luteinizing hormone (LH), which triggers the ovaries to release an egg. The body responds by producing more of these hormones to try and jump-start egg development. As you approach 50, your body stops responding to FSH and your menstrual cycle becomes shorter. Eventually the ovaries no longer release an egg every month. By menopause, there are few or no eggs left.

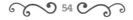 54

World's Oldest Moms

The amazing babymaking race has become something short of miraculous. Until recently, a 66-year-old Romanian, Adriana Iliescu, bore the title of oldest woman to give birth—to a daughter in January 2005 in Bucharest. But in December 2006, Spanish señora Carmela Bousada broke that record, delivering twin sons in a Barcelona hospital at age 67. She accomplished this feat by reportedly using donated eggs and in vitro fertilization (IVF) at the Pacific Fertility Center in Los Angeles. Vicken Sahakian, M.D., of the L.A. center, has said that he was "duped" by Bousada, who claimed to be 55 to qualify for the treatment. Medical ethicists have criticized these older moms, saying they probably won't live to see their kids enter adulthood, and are irresponsibly creating orphans. Wonder whether anyone said that to actor Anthony Quinn and novelist Saul Bellow, both of whom fathered children in their eighties?

Fertility Basics

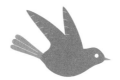

The Range of Normal

There's vast variation in women's cycles, and even the experts don't agree on the terminology that best describes a normal versus an abnormal menstrual cycle. But a 2007 study in the journal *Human Reproduction*, a collaboration between the OB-GYN departments at UCLA, the University of Sydney in Australia, and the University of Edinburgh in the United Kingdom, reported that a normal cycle can be anywhere from 24 to 38 days long with bleeding lasting 4 1/2 to 8 days. Yours doesn't fall within these parameters? Ask your doctor whether there's cause for concern.

Fertility Facts

Periods and Pregnancy

Researchers have been trying to figure out the characteristics of menstrual cycles that are most likely to result in pregnancy. A recent study of 470 women conducted by Emory University in Atlanta, Georgia, found that those with 30 to 31 day cycles and five days of menstrual bleeding were most likely to conceive. Shorter bleed times may reduce fertility because of a quick estrogen drop due to follicle deficiency or poor uterine lining buildup, the researchers suggest. But that's certainly not to say that only women with cycles this long, who bleed for this many days, will get pregnant. Any woman with regular cycles of any length—indicating regular ovulation—should be able to conceive.

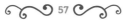

Short and Not so Sweet

Cycles that are routinely shorter than 24 days may indicate an underlying problem. For instance, an abbreviated follicular phase (the part of the cycle between menstruation and ovulation) may mean the egg won't have the time it needs to mature. A skimpy luteal phase (which begins after ovulation and generally lasts 10 to 16 days) may indicate that the body isn't producing enough progesterone for implantation.

A Painful Predictor

When it comes to our reproductive health, pain may not always mean problems. About 20 percent of women experience a condition known as *mittelschmerz* (German for "middle pain"). At midcycle, they feel a sharp pain or dull ache cramp on one side of their lower abdomen. It can last from a few minutes to a few hours, and sometimes for a couple of days, according to the Mayo Clinic. But mittelschmerz is rarely severe and shouldn't cause alarm. The pain, which occurs on the side whose ovary is ovulating, coincides with a follicle's rupture and egg release and may be due to ovary stretching or fluid released from the ruptured follicle irritating the lining of the abdomen. The condition rarely requires medical attention and can be controlled with over-the-counter pain relievers, if necessary.

Enormous Eggs

The human egg is the largest cell in the human body. And it's a beautiful sight to behold: Under the microscope, the maturing egg cell is a sphere surrounded by a radiant corona. At a size of 100 microns, or one-tenth of a millimeter, that's equivalent to the diameter of a single strand of hair. (Sperm cells, the other half of the reproductive equation, are much, much smaller. In fact, sperm cells are the smallest cells in the human body. How small are they? The answer is on page 183.)

The Temperature's Rising

Can less than 1 degree Fahrenheit make a difference? When it comes to fertility, yes. Countless women pop a thermometer in their mouths before getting out of bed every day to measure and chart their basal body temperature (BBT), a low-tech method of determining whether—and when—ovulation occurs. A woman's normal nonovulating temperature is between 96 and 99 degrees Fahrenheit. After an egg is released, it rises by about one-half a degree in most women. Because this heat-index increase is so small, you need a special basal thermometer to measure it. If you get pregnant, your temperature will remain higher through your first trimester.

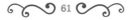

You're Beautiful When You're Ovulating

You've heard about the glow of pregnancy. Well, there's also a glow associated with ovulation. According to research, men perceive women as more beautiful when they're most fertile. In a study conducted at the University of Newcastle in England, 48 women were photographed during two different phases of their menstrual cycles. A group of men and women between the ages of 18 and 44 viewed the photos and chose the one they found more attractive. Most selected the pictures taken when the women were ovulating, preferring their more attractive lip color and size, dilated pupils, and softer skin color and tone. Interestingly, the women raters were more sensitive than the men to fertility's beautifying effect.

Fertility Facts

The Age of Motherhood

Over half of all births occur to women in their twenties, the peak childbearing years. But the average age of women giving birth to their first child has been shifting steadily upward, to 25 currently in the United States. That compares to an average age of 21 years for a first birth in 1970, according to a report from the Centers for Disease Control and Prevention. The report also shows that the average (or mean) age of mothers for all births rose from almost 25 to 27 years over the past three decades.

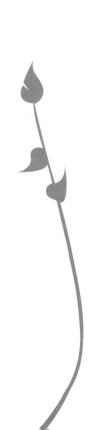

Fertility Basics

The World of Periods

Think about it: Most women menstruate once a month from the early teen years through the late forties or early fifties. That's a lot of cycles. In fact, for women in developed countries, it averages out to 450 over their lifetime, according to Richard E. Jones and Kristin H. Lopez, biologists at the University of Colorado, Boulder. In contrast, women in developing countries experience only about 160 periods during their lives. The difference appears to be due to the number of pregnancies a woman has and how long she breast-feeds. That's because during pregnancy women don't menstruate and the energy demands of breast-feeding usually delay the return of their periods. Women in underdeveloped countries may have more pregnancies than their counterparts in the developed world, and breast-feed each child for several years, a far cry from practices in the United States and other industrialized countries.

Fertility Facts

Four Million Moms

Who's having babies these days? According to the latest CDC data, more than 4 million women in the United States give birth each year, and more than 10 percent of those births are to teenage mothers. On the other end of the spectrum, just over 100,000 babies are born each year to women over 40. Between 2005 and 2006, the U.S. birth rate increased for women in their teens, twenties, thirties, and early forties. And as a result of this across-the-board increase, the total fertility rate (the estimate of the average number of births that a group of women will have over their lifetimes) is currently the highest since 1971, and the first time since then that the rate is above replacement level (the level at which a given generation can replace itself).

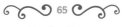

Unpopular Periods

Have you ever wished you could stop having periods (without compromising your ability to have a baby, of course)? You're not alone. A 2005 survey conducted by the Association of Reproductive Health Professionals found that 78 percent of women would be happier if they menstruated less frequently and 40 percent wished they didn't have periods at all. Certainly, there are disadvantages to the monthly flow. Women lose the iron and other nutrients found in the blood, and many experience pain with each period. But menstruation may be necessary to prepare the uterus for an embryo. In most other mammals, it's not necessary to prepare the uterus unless fertilization occurs, or their bodies absorb the lining of the uterus. In humans, the endometrium is so thick it can't be reabsorbed by the body, which is why it's sloughed off each month a pregnancy doesn't occur. So next time you're wishing you didn't have to deal with your period, just remember that the disliked and unappreciated period is a sign each month that the body's reproductive system is working . . . and ready for pregnancy.

Fertility Facts

Spend Half an Hour in a Cell

It's hard to imagine, but every human being on earth has spent 30 minutes as a single cell. That's because it takes approximately that long for the fertilized egg to divide for the first time. During the first two days, the fertilized egg grows to 2, then 4 cells, and by day 3, it's an 8-celled zygote, containing 23 chromosomes from the man's sperm and the 23 from the woman's egg. These chromosomes will determine eye color, hair color, and sex. The cells continue to divide as they're pushed along the fallopian tube, a kind of preembryonic dervish dance. Approximately four days after fertilization there are about 100 cells, and the zygote is now called a blastocyst. By day 6, the blastocyst is comfortably implanted in the uterine wall. And the rest, as they say, is history.

Fertility Basics

The Body's Built-in Ovulation Predictor

Every woman has an ovulation predictor built into her body, and it's absolutely free. Cervical mucus (CM), secretions produced in the nooks and crannies of the cervix (located in the neck of the uterus), change over the course of a woman's cycle. Regularly monitoring the amount and consistency of CM can help pinpoint when you have the best chance of conceiving. Using a clean finger inserted into your vagina or checking the toilet paper when you wipe yourself, you can check the sensation (dry, moist, or wet), color (white, creamy, cloudy, or clear) and consistency (sticky, smooth, or slippery).

When you're most fertile, the cervical mucus will feel slippery and may stretch up to several inches before it breaks. It will look thin and watery and be transparent like a raw egg white. This signals ovulation, and if all goes according to plan, sperm will be waiting when the egg is released.

Fertility Facts

The Odds Are in Your Favor

The least invasive potential cure for many fertility problems is a word easily overlooked: time. When both partners are under 30 or 35, waiting a little longer before jumping on the assisted reproduction bandwagon is a realistic option, notes Nanette Santoro, M.D., professor and director of reproductive endocrinology and infertility at Albert Einstein College of Medicine of Yeshiva University in New York City. Indeed, a major review of medical studies found that 90 percent of healthy fertile couples conceive within the first year of regular unprotected sex, and another 5 percent in the second year. Even couples who've received a diagnosis of unexplained infertility may want to wait before leaping into treatment: Within three years of the diagnosis, one in three will have a successful pregnancy with no treatment at all.

Fertility Basics

A Positively Fertile Mood

Our hormones affect more than just our fertility. Sex hormones have a job to do in virtually every part of a woman's body, and the major players (estrogen, progesterone, and testosterone) have some surprising additional powers. Before ovulation, estrogen levels rise, and that is related to positive feelings such as optimism and extroversion. Estrogen and rising levels of testosterone increase confidence, assertiveness, and competitiveness. After ovulation, estrogen and progesterone levels fall and progesterone, with its sedative properties, dominates. For some women, this ushers in a bout of the blues and they may become teary and emotional at the mere sight of a baby. As menstruation approaches, some women experience the physical symptoms of PMS (premenstrual syndrome) such as breast soreness and bloating. They may also have mood shifts, a result of the "crash" of sex hormones.

Fertility Facts

Testing, Testing

Ovulation prediction kits can tell you the days you're most fertile. Most work by measuring the level of luteinizing hormone (LH) in urine; the hormone is always present, but surges just before ovulation, triggering the release of an egg from the ovary. Tests typically detect the LH surge 24 to 48 hours before you ovulate. Some kits have you place a few drops of urine on a testing stick, while others have you hold the stick directly in the stream of urine. Still others have you collect urine in a cup, and dip a stick into it. Generally, a colored line means a positive result, indicating a good time for intercourse. More expensive electronic urine monitors, which provide a greater peak fertility window, are also available.

Secrets of Sweat and Saliva

Urine isn't the only bodily fluid that can predict ovulation. Some newer tests now use sweat or saliva to determine the fertile window. For instance, there's a watchlike device equipped with a sensor that measures the amount of chloride excreted in sweat. Increasing levels of chloride predict hormonal surges a few days before ovulation, giving you more notice than standard urine tests. Saliva-based microscope monitors, meanwhile, measure the levels of estrogen in electrolytes found in the saliva. You place a small sample on a lens, which is examined under a microscope after it dries. When estrogen levels rise—indicating a fertile phase—you see a distinct, fernlike pattern. The electronic version of this test makes interpreting the results even easier.

Fertility Facts

High FSH, High Hopes

When doctors want to determine a woman's ovarian reserve, they measure her level of follicle stimulating hormone (FSH). When it's high, it generally means she doesn't have a lot of eggs left in her ovaries. This typically is the case as a woman ages. But even younger women can have a high FSH level. And while it might mean they'll experience menopause early, it still may be possible for them to get pregnant. Even though the number of good eggs is diminished, the quality of the eggs that remain should still be good. Doctors say they've seen patients in their early thirties with significantly elevated FSH levels who have still been able to have babies.

A Nose for Pregnancy

Are things suddenly smelling stronger? That could mean it's a good time to try to get pregnant. According to Alan R. Hirsch, MD, a neurologist and psychiatrist, and neurological director of the Smell & Taste Treatment and Research Foundation in Chicago, Illinois, a woman's sense of smell becomes more sensitive around the time she ovulates. And the difference is pronounced enough for women to be aware of it each month. "If you're hoping to conceive a child, it's something to keep in mind," he says. When odors become more pronounced, make your way to the bedroom fast.

The Season for Having Babies

Have you ever wondered why there seems to be an explosion of very pregnant women during the summer? Your eyes aren't playing tricks on you. There's evidence that our fertility may be influenced by the seasons and that paying attention to this could influence your chances of conception. Over the past decade, July has been the most popular birth month, with August a close second, according to the U.S. Census. Some experts believe the summer birth rate bump is tied to fall holidays and family vacations, when couples spend more time together.

The Season for Making Babies

If most babies are born in the summer, it means they were conceived in the autumn: October, November, or December. One hypothesis holds that cooler fall temperatures make some couples feel more frisky after a hot summer. And the brisk, cool weather is also good for sperm production, which can be decreased in summertime.

Fertility Facts

The Real Birth Day

The Internet is rife with due date calculators and calendars. But no matter how you crunch the numbers, it's your baby who will decide when to make an entrance. And, these days, babies in the know are choosing Tuesday. According to the CDC, in 2004 (the most recent numbers available) the greatest number of births—13,045—occurred on a Tuesday, with Wednesday, Thursday, and Friday, not far behind. This trend held true for both vaginal and Cesarean deliveries, including repeat C-sections. The fewest number of births—8,496 and 7,501—were on Saturdays and Sundays, respectively. Perhaps women would rather miss a workday than a weekend day to give birth?

Fertility Basics

Dressing to Impress

Women may say they dress for themselves, but scientists have found there's another reason why they put on the glitz: They're advertising their fertility. Researchers at the University of California, Los Angeles, studied a group of young women and found that they often wore flashier clothing and jewelry when they were ovulating. Instead of pants, they wore skirts and showed more skin, notes lead researcher Martie G. Haselton, PhD, associate professor in the departments of communications studies and psychology. Talk about fertile fashionistas! Interestingly, Haselton has found that humans change more than their looks to advertise their fertility. In previous research, she showed that women were also more likely to flirt and look at attractive men around the time they were ovulating.

Fertility Facts

Hey Big Tipper,
I'm Ovulating!

In a study that probably gave male members of the research team a great deal of job satisfaction, researchers at the University of New Mexico in Albuquerque have found that lap dancers (women who work in strip clubs and get paid to "dance" while seated on men's laps) earn more money around the time they're ovulating. The 11 women with normal menstrual cycles averaged about $70 per hour during the most fertile phase of their cycle, $50 during the luteal phase (the part of the cycle between ovulation and menstruation), and only $35 while menstruating. The results indicate that women are somehow able to signal their fertility to men, although the how and why is still not well understood.

Fertility Basics

Chapter
3

The Fertile Lifestyle

You've heard of *Lifestyles of the Rich and Famous*? Well, far more important to anyone who wants to get pregnant is *Lifestyles of the Fit and Fertile*. How you live your life will affect the life you want to create. Now is the time to quit the bad habits that can impair your fertility, and embrace new ones that will help your body prepare for a healthy pregnancy. Some of the advice is good common sense, and some will surprise you.

Stay Calm for the Sake of Your Uterus

If you think your headaches and tight shoulders are the only physical manifestations of your super-stressed life, think again. Your uterus may be paying the price as well. A healthy uterus contracts about five times a minute, but stress can increase the frequency of those contractions, which can keep a fertilized egg from implanting in your womb. While you can't directly control the muscles that handle uterine contractions, you do have some power to relax them. By relaxing your voluntary muscles via yoga, meditation, or even a slow walk around the block, you cause your entire body to release its tension. When that happens, your involuntary muscles will relax as well.

Reduce Stress to Improve Your Chances

Science shows that reducing stress can directly and positively impact your chances of conception. In one study, published in *Fertility and Sterility* in 2000, researchers followed 120 women who had been trying to get pregnant for one to two years. One group participated in cognitive behavioral therapy, a second in a support group, and one group received no psychological treatment at all. After one year, women in the two groups receiving some psychological treatment had significantly higher pregnancy rates than those in the control group. In another study from Emory University in Atlanta, Georgia, private counseling sessions focused on destressing techniques seemed to help boost ovarian activity, a first step to conception. It's too simple to just say, "Relax and you'll get pregnant." But try to relax anyway.

The Fertile Lifestyle

Strike a Child's Pose

Yoga is good for the body, mind, and soul, say supporters. Now they may have new reason to promote the practice: it can improve fertility. A 2000 study from researchers at Harvard University tracked 184 women who were trying to conceive. The results showed that 55 percent of the women who completed a mind/body program like yoga got pregnant within a year, compared with only 20 percent in a control group. Many yoga facilities now even offer classes on "fertility yoga," combining traditional yoga postures with moves claimed to benefit both men's and women's reproductive health.

Fertility Facts

No Butts about It—Smoking Harms Fertility

You know smoking is bad for your heart, lungs, and skin, but did you know it's also bad for your fertility? Lighting up can prematurely age a woman's ovaries, and has been associated with an accelerated rate of atresia, or egg destruction. It also moves menopause up by roughly two years. Doctors know smoking reduces the amount of estrogen in a woman's bloodstream, and if you've smoked heavily for a long period of time, your chances of having genetically abnormal eggs are higher than for non-smokers. Smokers also have an increased risk of miscarriage, stillbirth, preterm delivery, and low-birthweight babies.

Smoking and the Second Generation

When you quit smoking now, you're not just helping to insure the health of your unborn child, but possibly the very existence of your grandchildren. Researchers have found that a mother's smoking before and after pregnancy can reduce her daughter's fertility by as much as two-thirds. According to a team at the Samuel Lunenfeld Research Institute of Mount Sinai Hospital in Toronto, Canada, the culprit might be a hydrocarbon chemical known as PAH, which is a pollutant found in cigarette smoke, car exhaust, and smoked food. When mice were exposed to this chemical before pregnancy or during breast-feeding, their female offspring were born with two-thirds fewer eggs than normal, limiting their future reproduction. Male fertility is affected by smoking, too, as previous studies have suggested that the male offspring of mothers who smoke have lower sperm counts.

Fertility Facts

See the Sunny Side of Life

Being exposed to at least 1 hour of sunlight a day may boost fertility. How? First, natural sunlight helps fight depression, a known fertility suppressant. Second, the pineal glad, which serves as the brain's "light meter," is part of the control system for reproductive hormones. If you don't get enough sunlight, the system won't be able to naturally regulate itself. So look on the bright side to feel more fertile.

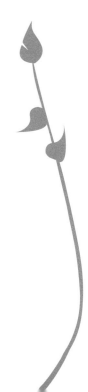

Take a Pass on Some Pain Pills

Doctors recommend women trying to conceive avoid nonsteroidal antiinflammatory drugs (NSAIDs), particularly during their most fertile periods. These medicines block prostaglandins, which are necessary for ovulation. Drugs in this class include ibuprofen (brand names include Advil, Motrin, and Nuprin); naproxen (brand names include Aleve and Naprosyn); and COX-2 inhibitors (brand names include Celebrex). While the occasional dose around the time of ovulation probably isn't a problem, a woman who consistently takes these drugs could see a negative effect on her fertility. Most doctors agree that the pain reliever acetaminophen (Tylenol) is a safe choice.

Fertility Facts

Marijuana Impairs Fertility for Both Partners

Whether it's you or your partner that uses marijuana, it's bad for fertility. A study at the University at Buffalo School of Medicine and Biomedical Sciences in New York found that the sperm of men who smoked marijuana had difficulty reaching an egg. The real surprise: the researchers say the same effect on sperm was noticed even if it was the woman who had smoked marijuana. The reason is that THC, the active ingredient in the drug, would be present in her reproductive fluids, as well, and would harm the sperm's biological pathway to her eggs. Abstaining from the drug for three months allowed men's healthy sperm to regenerate.

Past Abortions Don't Affect Current Fertility

The idea that a past abortion may be preventing pregnancy most often turns out to be all in a woman's head. No reliable evidence shows any connection between past first trimester surgical abortions or medical abortions (which terminate pregnancy through medication rather than surgery) and current or future fertility. If there were complications after the abortion, however, such as a post-operative infection or hemorrhage, there is a possibility that a woman's fallopian tubes could have suffered some damage. While many women feel guilt over past abortions, doctors say that in the majority of cases future pregnancies should not be affected. The message: get a checkup to rule out physical problems. And focus on the future rather than the past.

Be Careful
Of Chemicals

Substances found in some plastics and cosmetics could be harming women's and men's fertility. A subset of chemicals called phthalates are banned from many products in the European Union, but area still common in the United States. The substances, found in many soft plastics, cosmetics, and haircare products, can decrease sperm motility in men. Phthalates can be absorbed through the skin from sources like cologne, aftershave, and shampoo, inhaled as fumes from nail polish or hair spray, ingested orally through time-release medications or items stored in soft plastic bags, or even injected into the bloodstream through transfusions or IV fluids held in phthalate-containing bags. Another chemical used in plastics that has raised alarms, bisphenol A (BPA), causes chromosomal abnormalities in the eggs of otherwise normal mice. While researchers can't say for certain the chemicals would have the same effect on human fertility, there have been studies that show a link between BPA blood levels and miscarriages.

Steer Clear of Heavy Metals

While the link between heavy metals, such as lead and mercury, and negative health effects is well-established, men and women who are exposed to these substances while they're trying to conceive should be extra vigilant. Lead and mercury exposure has been linked to miscarriage, impotence, and reduced fertility in women, as well as lower sperm counts and decreased libido in men. If you or your partner is exposed to harmful chemicals in the workplace, the best option is to remove yourself from jobs where you come into contact with the substances. If that isn't possible, make sure you're protected by using gloves, masks, gowns, and other barriers.

Get Up and Dance!

Many cultures around the world have fertility rituals that include dancing, but most women in the Western world who are trying to conceive eschew late nights at night clubs. Dancing is a great way to get in the mood for babymaking. Beside being an intimate and fun experience with your partner, it also stimulates blood flow to the reproductive areas, which could actually aid in conception.

I Wear My Blue-Blocking Glasses at Night

Get ready to see the light: research shows that the body's pineal gland produces melatonin, a hormone necessary for reproduction, only during darkness. But thanks to our own wacky late-night schedules and electric lights, we interfere with our body's ability to produce this baby-boosting hormone. If you can't tuck in at sunset each night, however, there is a solution. You can wear special blue-blocking glasses for a few hours before bedtime each night to trick your body into thinking it's getting a few extra hours of darkness.

Fertility Facts

Needling Your Way to Pregnancy

While scientists continue to make groundbreaking discoveries, they're also finding that traditional practices for improving pregnancy rates are more than just old wives' tales. Case in point: research now supports the idea that acupuncture may have a positive effect in infertility treatments. A 2002 study in the journal *Fertility and Sterility* found that in vitro fertilization patients who received acupuncture just before embryo transfer were more likely to become pregnant than those who did not. In fact, 43 percent of the acupuncture group conceived, compared with 26 percent of the control group. Why did the needling procedure help with implantation? Researchers say acupuncture improves blood flow to the uterus. Want your partner to partake in the traditional healing therapy, too? Some evidence points to the idea that acupuncture can also improve sperm mobility and motility, as well.

The Fertile Lifestyle

Conception-Moon Over Miami . . .

You know what a honeymoon is, but what about a conception-moon? That's right: some couples who are trying to conceive now take a romantic vacation to help get them in the right mood. The idea, of course, is that time away from the hustle and bustle of everyday life will lead to relaxation, sex, and of course, pregnancy. One survey of over 1,000 members of a Web site who said they'd had fertility issues revealed that over 75 percent had taken a conception-moon while trying to conceive. But the most impressive stat was how many succeeded: Forty percent of the couples who said they'd vacationed to procreate came back pregnant. The most popular destinations? Las Vegas, Hawaii, and Florida.

Fertility Facts

Doc's Advice: Don't Douche

Staying away from these so-called feminine hygiene products is standard medical advice, especially for women hoping to conceive. Douches and vaginal sprays change the normal pH balance in the vagina and can cause inflammation and other allergic reactions that create a hostile environment for sperm. And that's not all—these products don't just change the environment in the vagina, but they can also wash away cervical mucus that smooths the way for sperm trying to make the precipitous journey to unite with an egg.

The Fertile Lifestyle

Chapter
4

Fertility Threats

Just as the right lifestyle choices can help boost fertility, poor choices can be reproductive hazards. Smoking, for instance, is bad for a lot more than your lungs. Some of these fertility threats are easy to avoid, and the benefits of making a lifestyle change to avoid them can be immediate. But many other fertility hazards— including common illnesses and conditions like diabetes or thyroid problems—can't be avoided, and have to be managed. Still other fertility threats, such as miscarriages, often have no explanation and are nearly impossible to avoid. But even here the news is good: The vast majority of women who suffer from miscarriages go on to have healthy pregnancies and healthy babies. So read on to find out about the fertility threats that can be avoided, the threats that can be managed, and the threats that may have to be endured . . . but can eventually be overcome.

Out of Bounds

If you regularly have pain with intercourse and excessive pain before and during your periods that doesn't improve with nonsteroidal anti-inflammatory medication such as ibuprofen, you may be suffering from endometriosis. The chronic disease, in which the tissue lining the uterus migrates to other pelvic structures—including the ovaries and fallopian tubes—affects 10 to 15 percent of women who menstruate. The body reacts to this misplaced tissue by forming scar tissue, which can prevent the fallopian tubes from picking up the egg and fertilization can't occur. The condition can be diagnosed with a laparoscopy, which involves inserting a small lighted tube through an incision, usually near the navel. This procedure can also remove or vaporize the growths, which some studies show can double the pregnancy rate. With more severe cases, in vitro fertilization can be helpful because it bypasses the tubes altogether.

Endometriosis Is Not a Fertility End

It's true that endometriosis is a leading cause of female infertility: 20 to 50 percent of women with infertility problems suffer from the disease, according to studies by the American College of Obstetricians and Gynecologists (ACOG). But endometriosis is not necessarily a bar to babymaking. Roughly 60 to 70 percent of women with the condition have no problem, according to experts at the National Institutes of Health. The determining factor seems to be how and where endometrial tissue lands in the body. Fertility is more likely to be affected if the reproductive organs are positioned badly or distorted from scarring. Endometriosis can also hamper fertility by interfering with egg development, causing scarring that can block the egg's travel to the womb, or making the uterus less receptive to implantation.

Fertility Threats

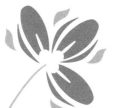

Silent STDs

Sexually transmitted diseases (STDs) are remarkably common: each year in the United States, there are about 3 million new cases of chlamydia, a bacterial infection, and 700,000 cases of gonorrhea. Many women have no symptoms at all, or the kinds of symptoms—such as fever and aches—that can easily be chalked up to something else, like the flu. What's more, symptoms may simply resolve on their own. But if left untreated, STDs can be a fertility hazard. In women, these diseases can cause fallopian tube damage or pelvic inflammatory disease (PID), a secondary infection of the uterus, fallopian tubes, and/or cervix. Ninety percent of PID infections are initially caused by chlamydia or gonorrhea, and 20 percent of women with PID experience infertility due to scarring. Surgery can usually remove the scar tissue and clear the path to pregnancy; when it can't, pregnancy can often be achieved with IVF.

Fertility Facts

Blocking the Path

Endometriosis and STDs aren't the only conditions that can cause pelvic scarring and block the path to pregnancy. Any kind of surgery to the pelvic or abdominal region can leave internal scars, as can past accidents and injuries. And women may not have any symptoms or any idea what's standing in the way of motherhood. The best bet: let your OB-GYN know your medical history and concerns. A peek inside via laparoscopy (lighted tube) or hysterosalpingogram (X-ray of the uterus and fallopian tubes) will show what's what. Many blockages can be removed with laparoscopic surgery (an outpatient procedure). In cases of severe damage, IVF can bypass the blockage to achieve pregnancy.

Too-Slow Thyroid Threats

A thyroid that's too slow (hypothyroidism) can throw a wrench in your reproductive plans, and you might not even be aware that this butterfly-shaped gland's speed is out of control. Symptoms of having an underactive thyroid include constipation, heavier periods, weight gain, a decrease in appetite, fatigue, and depression. Hypothyroidism can prevent ovulation by raising prolactin levels (a hormone involved in producing breast milk). It can also bring on a condition known as luteal phase defect, making it impossible for the body to build up a uterine lining to accept a fertilized egg. Simple blood tests can diagnose the condition, and taking synthetic thyroid hormones can set the speed to normal—and fertility.

Too Fast for Pregnancy

A thyroid that's too fast (hyperthyroidism) won't speed up your quest for a baby, but can sometimes prevent it. Symptoms of an overactive thyroid gland include frequent bowel movements, weight loss, irregular periods, insomnia, and nervousness. Hyperthyroidism can sometimes prevent ovulation, but a bigger problem is that once a woman with an overactive thyroid is pregnant, her metabolism may be so out of balance that the pregnancy can't go to term. After you're diagnosed with hyperthyroidism, medical treatments (including antithyroid drugs or radioactive iodine) will put the brakes on to restore normal function.

Fertility Threats

Cancer Patients Can

Cancer doesn't automatically mean an end to the hope of parenthood, just as it is no longer a death sentence. Even when the cancer affects the reproductive organs, there are fertility-sparing techniques that can sometimes be used to preserve reproductive function. When chemotherapy or radiation therapy threaten fertility, new techniques to save future fertility include egg or embryo freezing, ovarian transplant or transposition (in which ovarian tissue is moved to a safer spot in the body during radiation treatment), and drug-induced menopause (in which ovarian function is temporarily suppressed during cancer treatment, which seems to protect the ovaries during chemo). The result: more and more cancer survivors can now become biological parents.

Too Much of a Good Thing

Polycystic ovary syndrome (PCOS) is a leading cause of female infertility. Women with PCOS experience insulin resistance—the inability of the body to respond to and use insulin correctly. A chain reaction can result, upsetting hormone balances, causing the ovaries to overproduce male hormones such as testosterone, and disrupting normal ovulation. The first symptom is usually menstrual irregularities—long, irregular, or skipped periods. Other symptoms include excess facial hair (as well as extra hair on the chest, lower abdomen, or thighs), and acne and skin discoloration. What causes it? The condition may be partly inherited, since it tends to run in families.

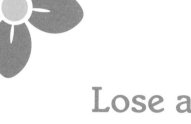

Lose a Little, Gain a Lot

The underlying cause of PCOS may be metabolic or inherited, but the condition can often be lessened or even eliminated with lifestyle changes. As many as 85 to 90 percent of women with PCOS are overweight, and in one study, nearly half of the obese women with PCOS who lost just 5 percent of their body weight were able to get pregnant without any medical intervention. Losing weight is key: even when women with PCOS still require medical treatment to get pregnant, they'll respond better to fertility drugs and have a healthier pregnancy at a lighter weight.

Take Control

Diabetes is not a threat to fertility in the usual way; it generally doesn't prevent conception unless the disease is way out of control. But untreated or badly controlled diabetes can cause damage to embryonic cells and cause a miscarriage so early—sometimes just days after conception—that women with the disease may think they're having trouble conceiving. The high blood sugar levels can prevent the fertilized egg from implanting in the uterus. Miscarriage rates among women with poorly controlled diabetes can be as high as 30 to 60 percent during the first trimester. But diabetes that's properly controlled months before conception should not stand in the way of a healthy conception and pregnancy.

Fertility Threats

Gut Reactions

Babies don't grow in their mother's stomachs, but what happens in the digestive tract can have a powerful impact on reproduction. Fertility problems are a little-discussed but increasingly recognized result of several serious gastrointestinal (GI) diseases affecting millions of American women. Women with two of these diseases—Crohn's disease and ulcerative colitis, known collectively as inflammatory bowel disease (IBD)—need to be particularly careful about how their disease is treated if they want to become pregnant. When the disease is controlled with medication alone, and not surgery, women stand a very good chance of achieving pregnancy. But surgery in the pelvic area seems to have a negative effect on fertility. So if you suffer from these illnesses and want to be pregnant some day, make sure your physician knows your intention before recommending treatment. The decision about what medication to take may be affected by your reproductive plans, too.

Fertility Facts

Shafted by Wheat

Celiac disease is a fairly common but often undiagnosed autoimmune disorder. Women with this disease have an allergic reaction to gluten, which is found in most wheat products, rye, barley, oats, and other foods. Celiac disease affects fertility in a roundabout way, by making it difficult for sufferers to properly absorb food. Unable to receive enough nutrients and vitamins, the hormones that stimulate the ovaries can be suppressed, preventing ovulation. Treatment for celiac disease is completely dietary: sufferers must avoid gluten and learn to balance nutrients properly. Once women with celiac disease follow a gluten-free diet, all symptoms of the disease will reverse, including problems with ovulation and conception.

Fertility Threats

Eating for 1 Before Eating for 2

It may not seem as if eating disorders—anorexia and bulimia—have anything to do with the reproductive system, but women battling those disorders may have a hard time conceiving. Women with anorexia may have a BMI so low that their hormone production is disrupted and they do not ovulate. Women with bulimia may appear to be normal weight, but may have severe nutritional deficiencies that can affect fertility. If not severe, these disorders may not be obvious to an examining physician. But if you suffer from an eating disorder and want to be pregnant soon, tell your doctor about the problem. You should get your weight—and your nutrition—in shape before you try to conceive.

The Shape To Be Pregnant

The uterus is often described as being about the size and shape of a pear. But some women may have been born with differently shaped wombs that they're completely unaware of until they try to have a child. In these cases the uterus may be heart-shaped (bicornuate), single-horned (with one fallopian tube), or divided (uterine septum), among other variations. These differences don't always cause problems with pregnancy, but when they do, they tend not to interfere with conception, but to cause repeat miscarriages. Treatment for a malformed uterus depends on the individual problem. Some women with severe cases choose to create embryos with their partners and have a surrogate carry the pregnancy.

HIV-Positive Moms-to-Be

It's no longer verboten for a woman who is HIV-positive to have a child. In fact, women with HIV can have a healthy baby with treatment during pregnancy and aggressive monitoring of the baby afterward. One caveat: women who harbor the virus that causes AIDS should not breast-feed their babies, as the virus can be passed on through breast milk.

Pregnancies Lost

Early pregnancy loss is so common that many obstetricians consider it a normal part of reproduction. Indeed, 20 percent of all pregnancies end in miscarriage, defined as the spontaneous end of a pregnancy during the first or early second trimester. Most occur within the first 12 weeks and some happen so early—before a missed period—that a woman may never know she was pregnant or that she miscarried. About 15 to 20 percent of miscarriages occur in the second trimester. "The majority of the time, a miscarriage is a random, isolated event and we can't pinpoint a cause," says Henry Lerner, MD, clinical professor of obstetrics and gynecology at Harvard Medical School. Some 20 to 40 percent of miscarriages are due to more tangible factors, such as infections, an abnormally shaped uterus, inadequate hormone production, immunologic problems, or environmental toxins. These miscarriages tend to occur later in the first trimester or in the second trimester.

And Pregnancies Found

It's devastating to lose a pregnancy, but the good news is that nearly all women who have had miscarriages go on to have healthy pregnancies and healthy babies. The chance that a woman will miscarry twice in a row is only 4 percent. Only 1 percent of women miscarry three times. Because the risk of recurrent pregnancy loss is relatively small, the standard medical protocol is to hold off on diagnostic testing until a woman has had three first-trimester miscarriages.

Fertility Facts

The Meaning of Multiple Miscarriages

Recurrent miscarriage has long been a medical mystery but new research is shedding light on factors related to early pregnancy loss. What's more, some cutting-edge tests and treatments are showing promise. Among them: pre-implantation genetic diagnosis, in which a cell from embryos created through IVF are examined for chromosomal abnormalities, allowing doctors to implant only healthy embryos; immunotherapy, in which antibodies extracted from the blood of donors are injected into the pregnant woman in an effort to protect the growing embryo; and blood-clotting treatments, subcutaneous (under the skin) injections of a blood thinner and daily doses of aspirin to ensure that the flow of oxygen and nutrients from the placenta to the fetus is not cut off by blood clots. The bottom line: having a miscarriage, or even two or three, doesn't mean you can't have a baby.

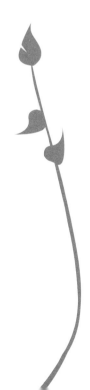

It's in the Genes

Most miscarriages are flukes and not your fault. In fact, the majority are due to a chromosomal error in the fetus, so your body may be acting in your own best interests by ending the pregnancy early. Chromosomes are tiny structures in each cell that carry our genes; we each have 23 pairs of them, one set from our mother and one set from our father. In a normal pregnancy, when a sperm fertilizes an egg, the chromosomes of the two cells fuse. But, sometimes the chromosomes get scrambled, which means the blueprints for fetal development are faulty, and the fetus dies within the first few weeks of pregnancy. Approximately 60 to 80 percent of miscarriages are thought to be due to this type of error. If you miscarry a second time, consider preserving the tissue you pass, if possible in a sterile saline contact-lens solution, and take it to your doctor to be sent to a lab for chromosomal testing.

Try, Try Again

Couples who have suffered a miscarriage want to know how soon they can start trying again. Many doctors recommend they wait until after a few normal ovulatory cycles or a couple of seemingly regular periods. That's because after a miscarriage, abnormal levels of hormones (such as progesterone) make it difficult for the endometrium—the lining of the uterus—to support a pregnancy. It can take two or three months for hormone levels to return to normal and for the body to start ovulating normally. Women undergoing fertility treatments can usually resume treatment after just one normal menstrual cycle. The medication may overcome any ovulation problems.

Chapter

5

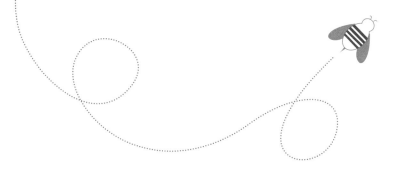

Diet and Nutrition

Before you can feed a baby growing inside of you, you have to feed yourself. And just as muscles and bones need the right nutrients to stay healthy and strong, the reproductive system has nutritional requirements, too. Many of the recommendations for "fertile eating" are exactly the same as the general dietary recommendations for overall body health. Others are more specific to reproduction. Read on to learn about the dietary habits that can help keep your reproductive system functioning optimally for maximum fertility.

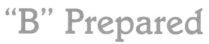

"B" Prepared

Getting enough folic acid, a B vitamin, is critical for pregnant women to help prevent birth defects in a developing baby. However, it's also vital that women get enough before pregnancy, since it's necessary for the very earliest stage of fetal development. The baby needs this nutrient to make the cells for his or her brain and bones, as well as organs and skin. The Recommended Dietary Allowance (RDA) for folic acid for all women, except those who are pregnant, is 400 micrograms. Best dietary sources are leafy green vegetables (especially spinach), citrus fruits, nuts, legumes, and whole grains. Since getting the daily requirement of folic acid through your diet can be difficult, many women depend on a supplement or multivitamin for help (for more information on folic acid supplements, see page 149).

Just Say "No" to Soy

Women trying to conceive should just say no to eating soy, at least around the time of ovulation. What's special about soy? It contains isoflavones, compounds that act like estrogen in the body. A study at King's College London found that one isoflavone, called genistein, can actually sabotage sperm as they swim in the female reproductive tract trying to fertilize the egg. So avoid consuming soy milk, edamame, miso, tofu, and any baked goods made with soy flour. Also be wary of vegetarian meat substitutes, as many are made from textured soy protein or tempeh, a soy product. Since some packaged foods may contain soy or soy protein, be sure to read food labels carefully.

Diet and Nutrition

Know the Facts About Fish

Regularly eating the wrong kind of fish, even a year before conception, can be harmful to your unborn child. Some fish contain high levels of mercury, which is toxic to a developing baby, and can take a year to leave the body. Women hoping to conceive within the next year should avoid eating shark, swordfish, king mackerel, or tilefish—the kinds of fish with the highest levels of mercury, according to the FDA. Also choose light canned tuna rather than albacore, which is higher in mercury. And be sure to check the safety of fish in local lakes, rivers, and coastal areas before eating it. As for other fish not on the high-mercury list, the FDA says eating up to 12 ounces of fish that are low in mercury weekly is safe. Shrimp, canned light tuna, salmon, pollock, and catfish are all low in mercury.

More Dairy Might Mean More Babies

Having twins can bring double the joy. And double the work, too. But according to a recent study, you can influence your chances of having twins by what you eat, or what you don't. Vegans, who eat no meat or dairy products, had only one-fifth the chance of having twins when compared to other women in a study conducted at the Albert Einstein College of Medicine of Yeshiva University in New York. Researchers compared the vegan women to vegetarian women who did eat dairy products, and to women who were not vegetarians. The dairy products may make the difference, researchers theorize, because of the growth hormones they contain from feed given the cattle.

The Antifertility Fat

Trans fats can damage more than your waistline and heart; they can also damage your chances of getting pregnant. According to researchers at Harvard University, the more trans fat a woman eats, the greater her risk of fertility problems. In fact, consuming just 4 grams of trans fat a day, which is less than the average American eats, can affect fertility. The researchers analyzed the eating habits of more than 18,500 married women who were trying to get pregnant, and had no known fertility problems. For every 2 percent of additional calories the women ate from trans fats, their risk of infertility increased by 73 percent. The researchers surmise that the trans fats somehow interfere with ovulation and may also increase inflammation in the body, which could affect fertility. To avoid trans fats, pass on products that contain hydrogenated or partially hydrogenated oils, and read labels carefully—food labels are now required to reveal any amount of trans fat over half a gram per serving.

Conception-Friendly Fats

Fat isn't always bad. Adding unsaturated fats to your diet can actually help improve your chances of conceiving because they reduce inflammation and insulin sensitivity, two factors that can disrupt hormone balance in the body. There are two kinds of unsaturated fats: monounsaturated and polyunsaturated. You can find monounsaturated fats in olive, peanut, and canola oils, as well as in avocados, cashews, almonds, and sesame and pumpkin seeds. Polyunsaturated fats, which include the omega-3 fats, can be found in fatty cold-water fish (such as sardines and salmon). Plant sources include flaxseed, walnuts, and vegetable oils including corn, sunflower, and safflower.

Bean-y Babies

You know you need adequate protein in your diet. But getting that protein from vegetable sources rather than meat can increase your chances of conceiving. Data from the Harvard *Nurses' Health Study* showed that adding one serving a day of vegetarian sources of protein such as beans, peas, or nuts provided some protection against infertility. In contrast, adding one serving a day of meat or poultry predicted a substantial increase in the risk of ovulatory infertility. Soy is a good source of vegetable protein, but try to limit your consumption to the less fertile times in your cycle (see page 123).

Fertility Facts

Fill Up on Fruits, Vegetables, and Whole Grains

Eating more complex carbohydrates like whole grains, fruits, and vegetables is the way to go when trying to conceive. Not only do they supply key nutrients, but eating them can also improve ovulation and your chances of getting pregnant. On the other hand, eating a lot of highly refined carbohydrates, such as white bread, will decrease your chances of conception. Highly refined carbohydrates increase your blood sugar and insulin levels, which in turn disrupt your hormone balance. The hormonal changes then affect ovulation cycles. To get complex carbohydrates in your diet, eat whole grains, beans, vegetables, and fruits. To find whole-grain products look for these ingredients on the label: whole wheat, stone-ground whole grain, whole-grain corn or cornmeal, oatmeal, whole or rolled oats, kamut, millet, amaranth, buckwheat, kasha, pearl barley, and brown rice.

Millet: A Fertility Wonder Grain?

Never heard of millet? See if you can find it in your grocery store. You may not be familiar with it, but fertility educator Julia Indichova has dubbed it the "fertility wonder grain." Millet is a whole grain, and it's wheat- and gluten-free. It helps balance blood sugar and insulin levels, thus keeping your hormones in balance. You can buy millet in cracked or pearled forms, as well as in flour. However, if you have thyroid problems, alternate millet with other grains; millet contains a compound that interferes with the production of thyroid hormones.

Do a Balancing Act with Your Food

Once you know what foods are good for you—and for your fertility—you also need to know how to balance them properly in your diet. The way you eat can help fight insulin resistance, which can compromise fertility by upsetting ovulation cycles and even increasing the risk of miscarriage. This condition especially affects fertility in women who are overweight or who have polycystic ovary syndrome (PCOS). To reduce the risk of developing insulin resistance, try to balance your meals and snacks by including one-third of the calories from protein, one-third from complex carbohydrates, and one-third from healthy fats. For protein, use lean sources such as salmon, turkey, or low-fat yogurt. Add complex carbohydrates such as whole-grain products, beans, or green vegetables. Avoid simple carbohydrates, such as white bread, because they trigger insulin response. Then include some monounsaturated or polyunsaturated fats, such as nuts, olive oil, or avocados.

Diet and Nutrition

Go Full Fat When It Comes to Dairy Products

Standard health advice is to look for low-fat or no-fat products, including dairy. But that advice changes when it comes to conceiving. One or two daily servings of full-fat dairy products seems to help protect against infertility. Consuming low-fat dairy products actually does the opposite. In a study of more than 18,000 women, researchers found that women who had one or more daily servings of full-fat dairy products were 27 percent less likely to be infertile than those who had less than one serving a week. However, women who ate two or more servings of low-fat dairy daily were almost twice as likely to be infertile. Just drinking one 8-ounce glass of whole milk daily cut the risk of infertility by 50 percent. Why the different results from the full-fat and low-fat products? Possibly because estrogen and progesterone in the milk attach to the fat globules. Skimming the fat skims off those hormones, leaving behind others that are not conducive to conception, such as some androgens, insulin-like growth factor 1, and prolactin.

Fertility Facts

Make Like Popeye and Eat Spinach (and Other Plant Sources of Iron)

A steak can be a good source of iron, but not for women trying to conceive. You can get iron from both meats and plant sources, but they're different kinds of iron. The iron from meat is called heme iron, but it's the iron from plants, called nonheme iron, that women who want to be pregnant need most. In the Harvard *Nurses' Health Study*, women who got most of their iron from nonmeat sources bettered their chances of getting pregnant. The women who got most of their iron from meat did not improve their fertility, and possibly even increased their chances of developing infertility. So be sure to include good plant sources of iron in your diet, such as spinach, red beans, and grain products (preferably whole grain, like brown rice or enriched cereals and breads). To help your body better absorb iron from the plant sources, have a vitamin C-rich food at the same meal.

Diet and Nutrition

Don't Over-Caffeinate

You're thirsty. What should you reach for? Well, plain water is best, but moderate amounts of coffee and tea are OK. The problem with coffee and tea is the caffeine they contain, which can stress your body, make you nervous, and affect your sleep, all of which adversely affect fertility. Most studies have found that moderate caffeine intake doesn't affect fertility. But a few studies have shown that high levels of caffeine may increase the risk of infertility or miscarriages. So most experts recommend keeping your caffeine intake to no more than 300 milligrams daily while trying to conceive. Keep in mind that one 8-ounce cup of coffee can have 65 to 120 milligrams of caffeine. One 8-ounce cup of tea can have 20 to 90 milligrams. Remember, there's always decaf!

Soda Savvy

Many soft drinks have 20 to 40 milligrams of caffeine per serving. So as long as you limit your consumption, your fertility shouldn't be affected. But experts say that even more than the caffeine in soft drinks, it's the sugar that may be the biggest potential problem. Sweet soft drinks can negatively affect blood sugar and insulin levels, a concern especially for women with PCOS, a common fertility-spoiler. So if you can't give up your soda habit, at least switch to sugar-free for now (ask your doctor if artificial sweeteners are safe during pregnancy).

Time to Grow Up

If you're planning to be a mother soon, one way to prepare is to give your diet a grown-up makeover. You're not eating for two yet, but you're eating to prepare yourself for pregnancy. That means if you still have childish eating habits of your own—too much junk food, soft drinks, fast food, or sugary sweets—it's time to switch to more mature eating habits. See a nutritionist if you need help with the makeover, or use your own grown-up judgment to banish empty calories and replace them with fruits and vegetables, whole grains, lean sources of proteins, and healthy fats that will provide healthy nourishment for you now, and give you a head start on healthy pregnancy eating soon.

Fertility Facts

Is Pre-Pregnancy Alcohol OK?

By now everyone (we hope) has heard that alcohol during pregnancy is a no-no. But what about before you're pregnant? The picture is a little fuzzier. Some experts advise that women abstain completely when trying to conceive because alcohol can alter estrogen and progesterone levels, and because most women won't know immediately that they're pregnant. Others say that occasional or moderate drinking before you conceive (meaning an occasional glass of wine) is OK, as long as you quit completely when you get that positive pregnancy test. If you want to play it safe, stop drinking while you're trying. But if you aren't ready to adopt a pregnancy diet yet, an occasional glass of wine is probably OK.

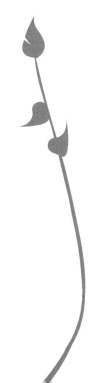

Wake Up and Smell the Cinnamon

Cinnamon can do more than flavor a dessert or cinnamon toast: it can also improve insulin resistance. Insulin resistance is a condition in which the body resists the efforts of insulin to regulate blood sugar. It's a risk factor for infertility, especially in women with PCOS. Women with PCOS typically have problems utilizing the insulin in their body. But in a recent study at Columbia University in New York City, women with PCOS who consumed 1 gram a day of cinnamon extract had significantly improved insulin resistance after eight weeks. Other studies have found that cinnamon may make cells more sensitive to insulin; it also may slow digestion, which would moderate a rapid rise in blood sugar after eating. So sprinkle some cinnamon on your whole-wheat toast or in your oatmeal every morning for a yummy treat, and a possible fertility boost.

Spoon Up
Some Cereal

One easy way to get the daily dose of folic acid in your diet is to eat a bowl of cereal that's been enriched with 100 percent of the RDA of folic acid. Read the label to see if the cereal has folic acid added, and if so, how much. Some brands that do contain 100 percent are General Mills's MultiGrain Cheerios®, Kellogg's® Special K®, Kashi's Heart to Heart, and Quaker Oatmeal Squares®. You can find a list of cereals with 100 percent of the folic acid RDA at http://cdc.gov/ncbddd/folicacid/cereals.htm.

Chapter

6

Vitamins and Supplements

Even the most well-intentioned eaters might have difficulty getting sufficient amounts of all the vitamins and minerals that are thought to promote fertility. That's where vitamins and supplements can come in. But with such a huge variety available, it's difficult to figure out what to take. Should you start taking a prenatal vitamin even before you're pregnant, or stick to one-a-day type multivitamins? Are there specific nutrient supplements that benefit fertility? What about herbs? While there are a lot of products available, there's also a lot of information to help you decide what would best supplement your diet to get your body baby-ready. Take a good look at your daily diet, and then read about the vitamins, minerals, and herbs that might give you an extra fertility boost.

The Mighty Multis

Women who are trying for healthy babymaking are usually savvy enough to pay attention to their diets, and are often already in the habit of taking a multivitamin supplement that is rich in the ingredients for a solid start to conception. Now, some doctors advise starting on a prenatal vitamin even before pregnancy, to help a woman's body get a head start on the added nutritional demands of conception and pregnancy. Another alternative: taking one of the many woman-specific multivitamins, which are often already fortified with many of the extra ingredients needed for healthy conception.

They Do a Body Good

Pop these pills for a fertility boost: a Harvard University survey revealed that women who had taken multivitamins and iron supplements were less likely to have ovulatory infertility than women who did not. One caveat: iron can be tough on some women's systems. If you develop nausea or stomach upset (and it's *not* morning sickness), speak up. Your doctor may have some advice ranging from switching supplement formulas to tinkering with your fiber and fluid levels.

Vitamins and Supplements

Supplemental Insurance: Folic Acid

Many women don't get enough folic acid from their day-to-day diets—a lack of which can be devastating to a developing baby. The American Dietetic Association recommends women of childbearing age take at least 400 micrograms in addition to what they would naturally get in a balanced diet to help prevent neural tube defects like spina bifida, as well as fetal growth problems, preterm delivery, and low birthweight. Since folic acid is especially crucial early on in pregnancy, most doctors now advise boosting levels as soon as women try to conceive. For those who find pills hard to swallow, consider this: many chewable children's vitamins contain the "magic number" of 400 micrograms of folic acid.

Fertility Facts

Chasteberry: an Ovulation Herb

Stanford University researchers discovered that women trying for pregnancy might benefit from natural over-the-counter supplements containing the herb chasteberry, which seems to help produce favorable changes in hormone levels and body temperature that could signal improved ovulation. The researchers speculate that the supplement may be especially helpful for women who struggle with irregular menstrual cycles that could be thwarting pregnancy efforts. One caveat: be sure your physician knows about all supplements you are taking. It's vital *not* to take chasteberry while undergoing in vitro fertilization, as it may actually reduce the pregnancy rate during that process. What's more, chasteberry is also not recommended during pregnancy.

Ironing Out
the Daily Diet

Get your "free" iron. That's the message sent by a November 2006 study in the journal *Obstetrics & Gynecology*. Researchers found that infertile women who consumed an average of 76 milligrams of iron each day—not just through supplements but in specific food sources—had a 60 percent lower risk of failure to ovulate than those who ingested the lowest amounts of iron. Because failing to ovulate is the second most common cause of infertility (after clogged fallopian tubes), this is big news. In the study, the women who consumed the most "free" iron—the kind found *not* in beef or pork but legumes, grains, fortified foods, as well as supplements—gained fertility protection.

A Modest Mineral

While folic acid and iron are sometimes referred to as the two most important pre-pregnancy vitamins and minerals, there's another mineral that plays an important role, too. Zinc, a trace mineral, is actually a reproductive all-star that plays a behind-the-scenes role in normal ovulation and fertilization in women. (Zinc is also an important fertility mineral for men; see page 197.) Most multivitamins and minerals contain zinc, although not all contain the entire amount recommended for women each day (8 milligrams before pregnancy, 11 milligrams once you're pregnant.) Check the label.

Put These Herbs on Hold

Some supplements claim to be fertility boosters, but others are best avoided when trying to conceive. A 1999 study in the journal *Fertility and Sterility* found that high doses of the herbs St. John's wort, ginkgo, and echinacea could damage reproductive cells and prevent sperm from fertilizing eggs. The real message is not to assume that something you buy without a prescription, or in an all-natural or health food store, is safe. Check with your doctor before taking any kind of herbs before conception.

Folic Acid Won't Make You See Double

While some previous studies reported a link between folic acid supplements and twin pregnancies, new research suggests there's no connection. Early studies that associated this vitamin with twinning looked at women undergoing high-tech fertility treatments, such as IVF. Women undergoing IVF frequently use vitamins and frequently have twins, so the results made it appear as if folic acid caused twinning. Later studies, including a 2003 study of almost a quarter-million Chinese women, and a 2005 study of 176,000 Norwegian women, showed no link between folic acid and twins in women who conceived naturally. So if you've been holding off on taking extra folic acid because you're trying to avoid twins, go ahead and take your vitamins.

Be "A"-Ware

Vitamin A is one vitamin that pregnant and pre-pregnant women need to be aware of: too much—more than 10,000 international units (IU) daily—can pose a danger of birth defects during early pregnancy. Most daily supplements contain 5,000 IU, but if women also eat many foods high in vitamin A (such as grains, cereals, and even granola bars), they might unwittingly exceed the safety limit. Read vitamin labels carefully. The form of vitamin A to be concerned about is retinol or retinyl. When vitamin A is included as beta-carotene, it's considered safe.

Beef Up Your Bs

While folic acid may be the most famous B-vitamin, it's not the only important one. B-12 deficiency has been implicated not only in causing repeated miscarriages, but also in infertility issues. Doctors theorize that B-12 deficiencies can cause changes in ovulation and negatively affect the ability of a fertilized egg to implant. Eggs and meat are prime sources of B-12, so vegans or strict vegetarians should consider supplements.

Vitamins and Supplements

An Ironclad Defense

If you think you don't need to worry about your iron levels until you're pregnant, think again: More than 20 percent of women of childbearing age already have low levels of iron in their blood, and a woman who has low iron *before* she conceives may find it especially difficult to replenish iron stores later on. Since research now suggests that adequate iron may help prevent miscarriages, many healthy experts now advise checking for anemia ahead of time. Even subclinical anemia (meaning there are no or few symptoms), which affects roughly 11 to 13 percent of American women according to the American Dietetic Association, could pose a danger.

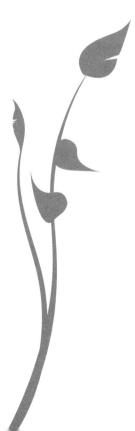

Check Your Vitamin Code

Be careful what you buy. Because vitamins haven't been approved as drugs by the Food and Drug Administration, the pills are treated as dietary supplements, which means they don't require standardization. Look for the USP label on any vitamin you choose. That's the stamp of approval from the U.S. Pharmacopeia, an organization that checks for safety and quality. Or check your own country's equivalent organization. To be on the safe side, many women involve their doctor or pharmacist in the decision of which brand to buy.

Can't Have Too Much Of a Good Thing

Worried that all the prenatal vitamins, B-vitamin supplements, and folate-rich foods you're eating could actually be too much? Don't fret. Because B-vitamins are water-soluble, they don't accumulate in fat tissue and are flushed out of your body on a daily basis. The flip side, of course, is that since your body excretes what it doesn't need, B-vitamins need to be replenished on a daily basis.

Herbs That May Help

Traditional Chinese Medicine (TCM) is gaining traction among Western physicians as a viable supplement to many modern medical practices. Women struggling with infertility have been turning to natural remedies for help conceiving. These remedies include licorice root (said to enhance estrogen production); wild yam root (a progesterone precursor that may be helpful for women with a too-short luteal phase); black cohosh, (for women with too much luteinizing hormone, or LH); and angelica or dong quai, which is used as a balancer for other herbs. As with many alternative treatments, the evidence for their effectiveness is largely anecdotal. Women should see a trained herbalist or naturopath before using these herbs, and should always tell their western medical doctors about all supplements they are taking.

Try Traditional Chinese Medicine

Beyond herbs, Traditional Chinese Medicine looks at the whole person and aims to bring the body into balance. Acupuncture is a commonly accepted branch of TCM, but the practice also employs herbal concoctions, tongue and pulse readings, and dietary recommendations as part of its healing methods. Some herbs used in TCM, such as saw palmetto, ginseng, and chasteberry, are familiar to North Americans. Saw palmetto is sometimes given to women who have symptoms of polycystic ovary syndrome (PCOS) since it is shown to reduce testosterone levels, a key player in the common infertility disorder. Ginseng is said to help balance the menstrual cycle, and chasteberry has a similar effect, particularly with women who are experiencing a lack of ovulation.

Be a Vitamin Vixen With Prenatals

Next time a tabloid catches a Hollywood starlet shopping for prenatal vitamins and exclaims she must be expecting, hold back judgment: the huge pills are actually a huge hit with stars looking for the latest beauty fix. The high levels of folic acid and biotin, a B-complex vitamin, are said to boost the beauty factor of hair and nails whether you're expecting or not. Folic acid helps in the growth of new cells, which makes it the perfect prenatal vitamin, but also means it promotes faster-growing, thicker strands of hair and stronger, less brittle nails. So both your hairstylist *and* your bouncing baby will be thanking you for your forward-thinking.

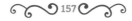

Chapter

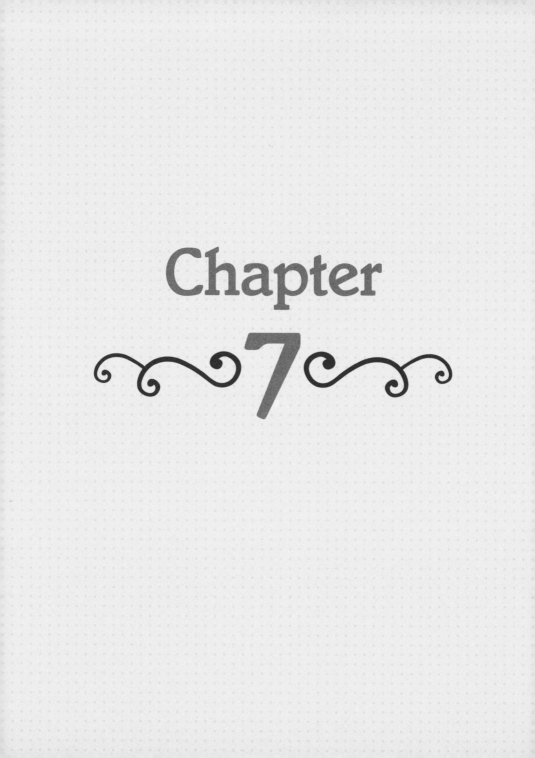

7

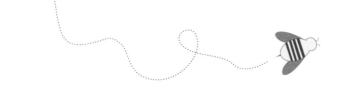

Fitness and Weight

You might think that the most vigorous exercise you need to do while trying to conceive is to have regular sex. But if that's what you're thinking (or hoping!), you're wrong. If anything, it's even more important to be fit and healthy while you're trying to get pregnant. Having a fit body at a healthy weight puts the odds in your favor for a quicker conception and a healthy pregnancy afterward. As for weight, well, there really is a body size that's optimal for fertility. Tipping the scales too high or too low can throw a wrench into your babymaking efforts. The good news: small changes can make big differences.

Work Out, but Don't Overdo It

Can you get too much of something good for your health? When it comes to exercise, you can. While exercise offers multiple health benefits, excessive or strenuous exercise can actually impede your chances of conceiving because it can lead to ovulatory dysfunction. When you're exercising strenuously, your body interprets that action as stress, and research shows that excessive stress can decrease fertility. But don't give up exercise entirely. Instead, moderate your exercise program to low-impact cardio, easy walking, swimming, yoga, muscle-toning, and resistance training while trying to conceive.

Fertility Facts

Eat Enough to Fuel Your Efforts

While many experts recommend against excessive exercise while trying to conceive, new research is showing that it may not be overexercising that causes fertility problems, but undereating. Athletes who don't consume enough calories to replace those burned in exercise won't have enough fuel left for other body functions. Their bodies will be forced to parcel out that limited energy to high-priority areas, leaving the reproductive system deprived of the fuel it needs to properly do its job. So if you're a serious athlete who's hoping to be a soccer mom some day, be sure to eat enough to take care of all your body's needs. A regular menstrual cycle is one important clue that your reproductive system is functioning normally.

Start Training for Pregnancy Now

Runners train for months to get ready for one marathon. So why not get in condition for the marathon of pregnancy? Make your exercise count toward the challenges your body will face once you're pregnant. Three types of exercise are recommended while you're trying to conceive: low-impact cardio (walking, swimming, fitness classes, water aerobics, treadmill, stationary bicycle, or elliptical trainer), muscle toning, and resistance training. The low-impact cardio provides high health benefits, with less risk of excess or injury. For muscle toning, work on building the core muscles of the back and stomach to strengthen them for the demands of pregnancy; good choices for this purpose are yoga or Pilates classes. Resistance training—using your own body weight or light weights—can also help prepare your muscles for the heavier load it will carry during pregnancy. By no means should you get into bodybuilding; if you use weights, don't exceed three pounds.

Fertility Facts

Keep Your Cool

Exercising can work up a sweat. But make sure you don't get too heated up. Raising your core body temperature above 102 degrees Fahrenheit can cause birth defects and miscarriages. Since you won't know you're pregnant right away, keep your cool while trying so that you don't accidentally expose your baby to excessive heat in its first few weeks. It would undoubtedly be awkward to bring a thermometer to the gym and frequently stop your workout to check your temperature. So instead, make sure that you exercise either indoors or outdoors in moderate temperatures, dress in cool clothing, stay hydrated, and don't overdo it. Avoid doing Bikram yoga or other similar classes that are held in overheated rooms.

It's Never Too Early

If you've been exercising regularly for at least a year, you've got a big head start on a healthy pregnancy. Regular exercise for a year before becoming pregnant can lower your chances of developing gestational diabetes. Continuing to exercise while you're pregnant can lower those chances even more. Why does gestational diabetes matter? Women who have diabetes have problems both in getting pregnant and staying pregnant. Plus gestational diabetes, which affects up to 6 percent of pregnant women, can contribute to miscarriages, premature births, and maternal deaths. But studies have shown that women who were the most physically active one year before their pregnancy had a 51 percent reduction in their risk of gestational diabetes. If they continued that activity for the first 20 weeks of pregnancy, their risk was reduced by 60 percent.

No Pain IS the Gain

Exercise offers benefits to your heart, bones, and mood. Turns out it can also help manage pain. Women with endometriosis, for example, may find that regular exercise can help them handle the physical pain of the condition, as well as the emotional stress of the fertility challenges that can result. Remember that exercise can't take the place of medical treatment for endometriosis, fibroids, or other painful and fertility-threatening conditions. But it can make handling them a lot easier.

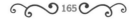

Belly Dancing for a Pre-Pregnant Belly

The tradition of belly dancing isn't about seducing men; in fact, in ancient times men weren't allowed to watch the shimmying. Belly dancing is a form of dance based on ancient fertility rites, and the movements actually target some of the muscles used in childbirth. Belly dancing while you're trying to get pregnant may not mystically make you pregnant. But it can provide an excellent aerobic and mid-section muscle-toning workout. And last but not least, what other exercise can you use to spice up your sex life? That alone might help you to get pregnant!

Fertile to the Core

Exercise programs targeting the body's "core" are popular for everyone trying to get fit, but these programs may be especially useful for women who are trying to conceive. Core strength (also called the "center," or in Pilates the "powerhouse") includes the deep abdominal muscles and the back muscles that support the spine. This part of the body is the key to a comfortable pregnancy and motherhood, as you will be hoisting around extra pounds for nine months and beyond. Think of all the extra pounds you'll need to carry around: first, while you're pregnant, around your middle; then, after delivery, a baby in your arms or perched on your hips. Having a strong core before you conceive may help you to avoid the back problems that so many pregnant women and new mothers suffer from.

"Om" Backward Is Almost "Mom"

There's a long history of belief in the fertility benefits of yoga. Beth Heller, codirector of Pulling Down the Moon, a Chicago studio that offers a special fertility program, explains that yoga enhances the life force within us, whereas modern fertility medicine practices can be life-draining. When Heller worked to develop a program of yoga poses aimed at improving fertility, she focused on the second chakra—or energy center in the body, located in the lower abdomen—which is the seat of creation. So far scientific studies haven't looked at how yoga improves natural conception rates, but there is some evidence that yoga—along with a program of emotional support, nutrition, and exercise—can help improve success rates in women undergoing fertility treatments. And, of course, it's great for fitness and relaxation.

Fertility Facts

Abs-olutely Right Now

No, it's not a waste of time to strengthen your abdominal muscles before you get pregnant. True, you might not see a flat stomach again until months after delivery, but getting your abs in shape before pregnancy can help you get through those nine months more easily. The abdominals are one of the muscle groups that get stressed most during pregnancy. If you strengthen them before you conceive, you'll have an easier time with the stresses on your body during pregnancy and an easier time getting in shape afterward. And you don't have to resign yourself to endless crunches to achieve strong abs. Exercises like boxing, stability ball toning, and even hula dancing can target the abs while you're having so much fun you don't notice.

The Thin and Thick of It

Many women's moods vary with what the scale says that day. As it turns out, so do your chances of getting pregnant. Experts estimate that a woman's weight, whether she is under- or overweight, may be a factor in up to 10 percent of infertility cases. Having either too much or too little body fat can confuse your brain, disrupt your hormones, and affect the release of eggs from the ovaries. So before you try to get pregnant, you may want to gain or lose a few pounds.

Fertility Facts

Know Your BMI (Body Mass Index)

Being either underweight or overweight can be a factor in infertility. But how do you know what weight is best? In this case, it doesn't really matter what you look like in skinny jeans. Instead, check your body mass index (BMI), and aim to be in the range of 18.5 to 24.9. A BMI of 25 to 29 is considered overweight, and 30 or greater indicates obesity. To help you find your BMI, the National Institutes of Health offers a BMI calculator on their Web site at www.nhlbisupport.com/bmi/ or an easy chart at the National Heart, Lung, and Blood Institute Web site (www.nhlbi.nih.gov/health/public/heart/obesity/wecan/learn-it/bmi-chart.htm). Prefer doing the math yourself? Take your weight in pounds and divide it by your height in inches, squared. Multiply that result by the number 703.

You CAN Be Too Thin

Being thin may help you fit into a smaller dress size, but it can also harm your chances of getting pregnant. It's estimated that about 12 percent of ovulatory infertility may be related to women being underweight. Being underweight can trick your brain into thinking that it doesn't have enough body fat and/or estrogen to support a pregnancy. As a result, the brain doesn't send enough GnRH (gonadatrophin-releasing hormone) to the pituitary gland. In turn, the pituitary doesn't send out the luteinizing and follicle-stimulating hormones that stimulate the follicles to release eggs. An analysis of data from the *Nurses' Health Study* at Harvard University found that underweight women with a BMI lower than 19 took four times longer to get pregnant than women in the normal range of 19 to 24. So what can you do? Sometimes gaining as little as 5 pounds can be enough to return your menstrual cycle to normal.

Fertility Facts

A High BMI Can Mean a Low Chance Of Conceiving

Being overweight can affect more than your vanity. It can also negatively affect your chances of getting pregnant. An estimated 25 percent of ovulation-related infertility may be due to excess weight. Why? Having too much body fat gives your body higher levels of estrogen. When estrogen levels are low, your brain is cued to signal hormones that trigger the release of new eggs from your ovaries. But the higher levels of estrogen can keep the brain from sending out those hormones. Being overweight also increases the odds of developing polycystic ovary syndrome (PCOS) and insulin resistance, conditions that can negatively affect your chances of conceiving. Insulin resistance is a condition in which your cells resist the efforts of insulin to distribute glucose. PCOS is a condition in which ovarian follicles fail to rupture and release eggs, resulting in the formation of cysts. What can you do? Losing as few as 10 pounds could improve you chances.

Fat Eggs?

Excess weight may throw hormones out of whack, but scientists are finding out more reasons why being overweight can hamper a woman's ability to get pregnant. In Australia, researchers at the University of Adelaide found that when mice consumed a diet high in fat, the eggs stored in their ovaries were damaged. Those eggs were not able to become fertilized and develop into healthy embryos. And in Spain, researchers at the University of Valencia found that the endometrium (the uterine lining) may be affected in overweight women, making it difficult for fertilized eggs to implant. Losing excess weight, say the researchers, will give women the best chance of successful conception and pregnancy.

Now's Not the Time For Crash Diets

A house depends on having a good foundation, and so does your pregnancy. Build that foundation by eating wisely long before you get pregnant. Ideally you should begin eating healthfully up to a year before you conceive. What does eating healthfully mean? Get at least twenty foods a week from the food groups in the food pyramid: grains, preferably whole-grains; fruits and vegetables; meat or vegetarian meat sources such as beans, milk, or dairy products; and healthy fats, such as nuts and olive oil. To learn more about the food pyramid, visit the Web site at www.mypyramid.gov.

If you need to lose weight, aim to do it before you start trying to conceive. Or check with your physician to make sure that your pre-pregnancy diet contains all the nutrients your body will need to conceive. (Once you're pregnant, dieting to lose weight is an absolute no-no because your growing baby needs sufficient nutrients from the food you eat.)

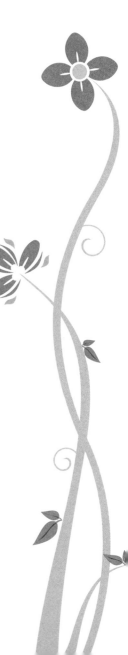

The 10-Pound Difference

Being overweight can cause problems in conceiving. But for some women, especially those with polycystic ovary syndrome (PCOS), losing just 5 percent of body weight can make the difference. For example, for a woman who weighs 200 pounds, losing just 10 could help improve the chance of conception. PCOS is the most common cause of women not being able to conceive, affecting approximately one in ten women of childbearing age. As many as 85 to 90 percent of women with PCOS are overweight. For many of these women, diet and lifestyle changes that lead to weight loss— even small to moderate weight loss—can restore normal ovulation and let conception occur.

Lose Weight Now for Your Future Family

You can take steps now, even before you're pregnant, to make your children healthier. A recent study found that women who were overweight when they conceived had children who grew up overweight. The study looked at children who were heavier than 95 percent of their peers at ages 3, 5, and 7. The researchers found that these children's mothers were likely to have been overweight or obese at least a month or two before they became pregnant. The take-home message is lose the weight before you get pregnant.

Fitness and Weight

Chapter

8

Just for Men

When it comes to making a baby, it obviously takes two, and men are equal partners in the process. Male fertility is just as much a factor in a successful conception and is equally to blame when things don't go as smoothly as planned. While many of the same lifestyle factors act as fertility boosters—or threats—in men and women, there are also things that are specific to men. For instance, since the male reproductive equipment is mostly outside the body, it can be more vulnerable to environmental threats such as heat, pressure, and trauma. On the other hand, women ripen a single new egg approximately every month, while men manufacture millions of sperm daily. You might think that means there's lots more room for error, but that's not really the case. Find out what's important for *him* to know when he's hoping to become a father soon.

Information Storage

A single sperm cell may be responsible for half the genetic material of a future human being, but all that information is crammed into a very small package: the sperm cell is the smallest cell in the human body. The head of a mature sperm cell is only about 5 microns wide. How big is that? Well, 1 micron is 1/100 the width of a human hair. Put another way, if a sperm cell were the size of a pinhead, a man would fill a room with his ejaculate! (How does the size of the human egg compare? See page 60.)

Shorter Sperm Cycle

The life cycle of sperm cells may not be as long as once thought. Scientists used to think that sperm lived from 70 to 90 days after being produced, but new research at the University of California, San Francisco, suggests the sperm life cycle is actually just about 42 days long. The shorter life span isn't all bad news for couples. The findings mean that male infertility treatments may work more quickly than previously thought.

Not Just a
One-Hit Wonder

Experts used to think a woman could get pregnant if she had intercourse before, during, or right after ovulation. Now doctors know that pregnancy is most likely when couples have sex in the five days *before* ovulation, or on the day itself, but not after. When an egg is released from the ovary, it's only receptive to sperm and able to be fertilized for about 12 to 24 hours. But according to Philip E. Chenette, M.D., reproductive endocrinologist at Pacific Fertility Center in San Francisco, California, sperm can remain viable and mobile in the female reproductive tract for days after intercourse. So the smartest conception plan is to have sperm ready and waiting when the egg is released.

How Many Sperm Can Fit in a Teaspoon?

A typical male ejaculate contains about a teaspoon of semen, which contains 250 million sperm—a staggering number! But of all those millions of sperm, about 50 to 100 actually reach the fallopian tubes after sex. In typical synchronized fashion, the sperm swim and worm their way through the vagina in the hopes of making it to the fallopian tubes. Most of the sperm release an enzyme that helps clear the pathway to the egg, so that just one sperm can penetrate it and begin fertilization. From 250 million to one—what incredible odds!

Men: Don't Have Too Much Fun Alone

When men are trying to become fathers, frequent masturbation around their partner's fertile period can temporarily reduce the sperm count and lower the odds. But occasional masturbation is not a concern. Unlike women who rely on a narrow conception window as an indicator to fertility, men have a 24/7 sperm factory at work. Most couples who are trying to conceive are advised to have sex every other day around the time of ovulation. Men who masturbate on the "off" days probably won't lower their sperm counts enough to affect conception.

Fertility Facts

Sperm, Sperm, Sperm . . . and Eggs

From the moment men hit puberty, the average male produces 50,000 to 60,000 sperm per minute. Yes, *per minute*. That's about 1,000 per second, faster than a machine gun spitting out bullets. All those millions of sperm cells are either ejaculated or reabsorbed by the body.

Sperm Ingredients

Men who enjoy chili peppers, garlic, and other spicy foods for dinner may wonder if those gustatory delights will affect their chances for babymaking later that night. No worries, dietary preferences don't have any appreciable effect on sperm. Male ejaculate is mostly made up of citric acid and sugar, and contains only 5 to 7 calories per teaspoon. In fact, the sperm cells themselves are only a small part of the fluid that's boosted with ingredients for fuel; the ejaculate contains just 1 percent of sperm by mass.

Fertility Facts

Shape Up, Stay Cool

Exercise is a great way for men or women to get their bodies into shape before having a baby. But in order to avoid potential male fertility and potency problems, men should make sure to keep their testes cool. Sperm production requires a body temperature between 94 and 96 degrees Fahrenheit. Even a temporary spike in temperature can interfere with conception. Marc Goldstein, M.D., director of the Center for Male Reproductive Medicine and Microsurgery at the Weill Medical College of Cornell University in New York City, recommends that men stay away from saunas, hot tubs, and steam baths while trying to conceive.

Accurate to
1 Degree

Warming up a man's scrotum can be a recipe for male infertility and potency problems. That's why men are advised to avoid wearing tight shorts or jock straps. Even a 1 degree Fahrenheit increase in body temperature can be enough to stop sperm production and kill off any remaining cells already produced. That's why Mother Nature put the male reproductive organs outside the body: to keep them cool. Too-tight shorts and nonbreathing fabrics can increase scrotal temperatures. Men should wear clothing that fits loosely and allows the testicles to hang free.

Men Hear the Clock Ticking, Too

Ladies, it's official: men hear the sounds of the baby clock going tick-tock, too. Harry Fisch, M.D., director of the Male Reproductive Center at Columbia University Medical Center of New York Presbyterian Hospital in New York City, shocked the medical community in 2004 when he suggested that biological clocks apply not only to women, but to men as well. Dr. Fisch points out that men in their mid-to-late thirties often see a sharp increase in the incidence of genetic defects in their sperm. And a series of studies conducted in Britain, the United States, and Sweden concluded that children born to older fathers face an increased risk of autism, schizophrenia, dwarfism, Down syndrome, and other genetic and chromosomal problems. Need further proof? A study at INSERM, the French National Health Institute, found that male fertility could decrease by up to 70 percent after age 40. The study also found that not only does the volume of sperm decrease as men get older, but the sperm also turn more sluggish. The message is men shouldn't delay fatherhood too long, either.

Soy Can Be a Sneaky Enemy

Soy can be a healthy source of protein. But it's not healthy for men's sperm. Soy contains a natural form of estrogen which can cause poor sperm quality in men who eat a lot of it. Even if you're not a vegetarian who relies on tofu and soy meat substitute for protein, you may still be getting more soy in your diet than you realize. Soy is included in many common packaged and processed foods. So while you're trying to conceive, be sure to read food package labels and to ask if soy products are in a dish when you eat out.

Eat Vegetables (and Fruit)

Spinach made Popeye stronger, and now, research shows that eating vegetables can make a man's sperm stronger, too. The more fresh produce a man eats, the better able his sperm is to fertilize an egg. Researchers at the University of Rochester in New York asked both infertile men and men who had fathered children in the past year to record their eating habits. They found that the men who had eaten the least fresh produce had the lowest sperm motility. An overwhelming 83 percent of the infertile men ate very few fruits and vegetables, compared to only 40 percent of the fertile men. Fresh fruits and vegetables contain antioxidants that help protect sperm from damage. Two antioxidants in particular, glutathione and cryptoxanthin, which are found in brightly colored produce, are especially helpful. So men, remember the food pyramid and try to eat five daily servings of fruits and vegetables—especially brightly colored ones such as carrots, tomatoes, blueberries, and oranges.

Just for Men

Think Brazilian

Nuts provide healthy fats. But one kind of nut also provides an antioxidant that's especially fertility-friendly. Brazil nuts are high in selenium, which helps prevent cell damage and is helpful for sperm function and fertility. There are selenium supplements, but some studies have shown they may be harmful to men who have diabetes or who are at risk of developing the disease. Until more studies are done, researchers suggest that diabetics not take selenium supplements, but get the nutrient through their diet. A man can get the recommended amount—55 micrograms a day—from just a few Brazil nuts. In fact, just 1 ounce of dried Brazil nuts provides 780 percent of the daily value for selenium, so the nuts should be eaten sparingly.

Yes, Men Have to Take Their Vitamins, Too

Even if a man eats a healthy diet full of fruits and vegetables, there are still some vitamin and mineral supplements that can help boost fertility. Vitamins C and E, selenium, and coenzyme Q-10, for instance, have all been shown to help fertility. Vitamins C and E are antioxidants that can help protect sperm from damage. Selenium, another antioxidant, has been shown to improve sperm function and fertility. (However, if your man is diabetic, he should likely avoid selenium supplements—see facing page) Yet another antioxidant, the vitamin-like substance coenzyme Q-10, is naturally found in the testes and improves sperm motility.

Spoon Up Some Tomato Soup

Perhaps one of the tastiest ways to increase male fertility is by eating a bowl of tomato soup. Tomato soup's special fertility ingredient is the carotenoid lycopene, present in tomatoes. Lycopene is actually absorbed better once tomatoes are processed, as in tomato soup, juice, and sauce. Men naturally have lycopene in the prostate gland and other organs, but men who are infertile often have low levels of the substance. In one recent study, researchers at the University of Portsmouth, England, had a group of six healthy men consume a can of tomato soup daily for two weeks. Levels of lycopene in the men's sperm rose between 7 and 12 percent.

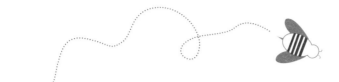

Cut Down on Coffee

Guys, cut down on your java intake for your future children's sake. Research shows that drinking even average amounts of coffee can increase damage to DNA in sperm. And evidence is growing that this damage can increase the risk of defects and mutations in children. How much coffee is safe to drink? Try to keep it to two cups daily.

An Exception to the Cut-Down-on-Coffee Rule

For men who've been diagnosed with sluggish sperm (low sperm motility), caffeine can act as a stimulant for those little guys, too. Sperm motility is the strength with which sperm swim toward the egg to fertilize it; when motility is low, sperm may not have the speed and power to reach the egg. But drinking coffee increased that motility in a Brazilian study of 750 men, thus increasing their fertility. If you think your sperm could use a pick-me-up, ask your doctor how much coffee would give them a caffeine boost without damaging their DNA.

Fertility Facts

Oysters and Pumpkin Seeds

The mineral zinc is important for testosterone and semen production. And wouldn't you know it, but the food that's often purported to be an aphrodisiac, oysters, is brimming over with zinc. Just two cooked oysters can give a man enough zinc to meet his daily requirement. The mineral is also found in beef, lamb, pork, shellfish, spinach, and pumpkin seeds. Also, there might be something to that oysters-as-aphrodisiac theory after all. Scientists have found that oysters, along with mussels and clams, have high levels of two amino acids that help increase levels of sex hormones. The levels of these amino acids are highest in spring when the shellfish are breeding themselves. Cooking reduces the quantity of the amino acids, so it's best to eat the oysters raw.

Meet Carnitine

A little-known nutrient called carnitine is found in most of the cells in your body and in seminal fluid, where it aids in sperm count and movement. Studies have shown that taking carnitine supplements can improve sperm quality and motility. But unless you're a vegetarian, you can easily get carnitine from food. The word "carnitine" comes from the Latin word for flesh, *carnus*, because it's mainly found in meat. A 4-ounce steak has 56 to 162 milligrams of carnitine compared to a 4-ounce chicken breast, which has only 3 to 5 milligrams. A cup of whole milk provides 8 milligrams.

Stay Away From Certain Supplements

Just as for women, some vitamins and minerals can act as big fertility boosters, while others can inhibit your efforts. For men, doctors say it's possible that the herb saw palmetto has a negative effect on fertility, since it lowers levels of the male hormone dihydrotestosterone, which is thought to be important for sperm production and ejaculation. As with any vitamins, minerals, herbs, or supplements, make sure your physician knows what you're taking, especially while you're trying to conceive.

Put Out
That Cigarette

Smoking cigarettes is already one of the worst things someone can do to his or her health. But men can add sperm damage to the list of health hazards from smoking. Researchers at the University at Buffalo in New York compared sperm from men who were smokers and non-smokers. The sperm from the smokers had more difficulty fertilizing an egg. In a Danish study of more than 2,500 men, researchers found that sperm concentration, volume, count, and motility were negatively affected by smoking. Nonsmokers had a 19 percent higher sperm concentration than did the smokers. If that news isn't persuasive enough to make you quit, consider this: cigarette smoking also reduces blood flow to the penis, possibly leading to impotence. It also decreases male sex drive and satisfaction. Time to butt out for sure!

Fertility Facts

Don't "Stone" Your Chance for Fatherhood

Smoking marijuana can "stone" a man's sperm, damaging it in several ways. Scientists at the University at Buffalo in New York examined 22 men who had smoked marijuana about 14 times a week for at least five years. They found that the men's sperm was damaged, racing too quickly to reach an egg, then becoming "burned out" and less effective once they arrived. The men also had significantly reduced sperm counts and amounts of seminal fluid. So when you're trying to conceive, just say "no."

Skip the "Love Drugs"

Ah, the mood is right and you've decided to pop a Viagra to make the experience last. But if you're planning for a baby, think twice before popping that pill. At Queen's University in Belfast, Ireland, Dr. David Glenn and a team of researchers found that a single 100 milligram dose of Viagra can prematurely activate the acrosome on the head of the sperm. What's the acrosome? It's the little sac of enzymes that makes the outer membrane of the egg dissolve a little so that the sperm can penetrate the egg. If the acrosome pops off too soon, it won't do its duty at the right time. If you're planning to become a Daddy soon, you might want to ditch the drug for a while and let nature take its course.

Get Needled

The art of Traditional Chinese Medicine (TCM) has been around for centuries. TCM studies the whole person—physical, mental, and emotional—and aims to bring the body back into balance. The body's energy—or chi—runs along pathways in the body called meridians. When that energy is blocked or unbalanced, illness can occur. Now there's new research that says acupuncture can help sperm mobility and motility. To support the claims, a research team at Christian-Lauritzen-Institut in Ulm, Germany, studied the sperm quality of 40 men who were considered infertile, with unexplained sperm abnormalities. Twenty-eight of the men received five weeks of acupuncture treatment, while a control group of 12 men received no treatment. Scientists found the group that received acupuncture treatment reduced the number of structural abnormalities in sperm, and increased the total number of normal sperm. Over the course of the three-year study, more than 20 percent of the participants who received acupuncture were able to become fathers.

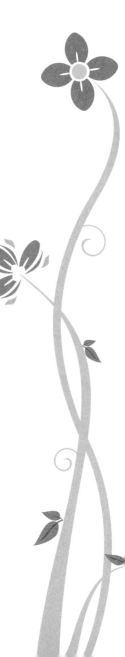

Porn for Parenthood?

Famed football legend Vince Lombardi was referring to sports when he said, "Winning isn't the most important thing; it's the only thing," but researchers say his quote may hold true for the reproductive race, too. A study at The University of Western Australia in Perth has shown that men produce better sperm samples with a higher percentage of motile sperm after looking at images that depict "sperm competition." Translation: Sperm samples improved after men looked at pornographic pictures of heterosexual encounters. The implication of the study is that humans, like many other animals, produce better sperm in situations where they observe competition for reproductive access to a desirable female. Now couples trying to conceive have another reason to watch something steamy together and enjoy the benefits.

Fertility Facts

Brush Your Way to Better Fertility

Your dentist was right about developing a proper flossing-and-brushing routine. Besides fresh breath and pearly whites, good oral hygiene can actually improve male fertility. Poor oral hygiene and bacterial infections associated with gum disease can infect a man's semen by spreading through the circulatory system, says Robert H. Gregg II, D.D.S., a California dentist and laser clinician. Even though antibiotics are a great way to knock out the infections, Dr. Gregg says the best way to avoid future problems is laser treatment of the damaged gums. Dr. Gregg, who is also a certified laser educator with the Academy of Laser Dentistry, points out that after the laser treatment, formerly subfertile men can show improvements in sperm quality and density.

Just for Men

A Toast to Moderation

Alcohol may offer some health benefits (red wine, for instance, has been shown to reduce the risk of heart disease), but consuming large amounts of wine, beer, or hard liquor can hamper male fertility. Marc Goldstein, MD, director of the Center for Male Reproductive Medicine and Microsurgery at Weill Medical College of Cornell University in New York City, recommends that men limit alcoholic beverages to no more than two drinks twice a week. Too many libations can affect the quality of sperm and even lower the level of testosterone that's necessary for sperm production. Alcohol can also cause breakages in the sperm's DNA that can be passed to offspring.

An Equal-Opportunity Fertility Hazard

Sexually transmitted diseases can be a fertility hazard to both sexes. Infections like chlamydia and gonorrhea have been known to cause infertility in women, and now research is demonstrating negative effects on sperm, too. Chlamydia rarely has any symptoms, but left untreated it can result in scarring in the ducts of the epididymis, vas deferens, and ejaculatory glands. When Swedish researchers tested 244 infertile couples for antibodies to chlamydia, they found that the couples in which either partner tested positive for the antibodies—the result of a past or current infection—had decreased pregnancy rates.

Post-Workout Shower Power

After you've worked up a good sweat in a jog or tennis game, make sure your post-workout activities are fertility-friendly: i.e., give your private parts a proper cool-down. Take a nice cool shower and then let your testicles hang down and free for a while. Yes, that might be difficult if you fit your workouts into office lunch hours, but at least try to change into loose, cool clothing that breathes. Or think about changing your routine so you're exercising after work instead.

The Season of Love

The hot summer months may be a great time for family vacations and trips to the beach, but they may not be a great time to conceive. There's evidence that fertility is affected by the seasons, and that high outdoor temperatures could have a negative impact on sperm. A 1994 study in the medical journal *Annals of the New York Academy of Sciences* found that there is a definite decrease in conceptions in the United States during July and August, especially in the Southern states. Medical experts believe this is linked to higher temperatures decreasing sperm count. According to Scott Slayden, MD, reproductive endocrinologist with Reproductive Biology Associates in Atlanta, Georgia, men with low sperm counts can experience a worsening effect of their condition during the summer months.

Take the Pressure Off

Cycling is great exercise, but it can be bad for a man's chances of getting his partner pregnant. The problem isn't the exercise itself, but the bicycle seats. Many seats, especially older ones, are designed so that when a man sits on them, they press against his perineum, the nerve- and artery-filled area between the rectum and scrotum. If a man sits that way for more than a few hours a week, the pressure can result in numbness or reduced blood flow to the genitals. For some men, that can mean losing the ability to achieve or maintain an erection. While the impairment is usually temporary, some serious cases can require surgery. Cycling isn't the only culprit. Men can also develop numbness from rowing in boats or machines (although this sport poses far less of a risk than cycling). If you really want to ride a bike, make sure your seat doesn't have a "nose" in front, and is designed to accommodate your reproductive equipment. If you can't switch seats, at least limit your riding to three hours weekly, and angle your seat properly to lessen the pressure on the perineum.

Fertility Facts

Avoid Traumatic Experiences

Contact sports are hard enough on a man's body, but they pose a special threat to the testicles. Sports such as football, soccer, martial arts, and boxing can result in traumatic blows to the groin, possibly affecting sperm production and fertility. At worst, a bad blow can even rupture the testicles, causing bleeding into the scrotum. In that case, the sperm is exposed to the body's immune system, which may begin attacking it. If you and your partner are trying to conceive, consider taking time off from any risky sports. If you still want to play, wear a hard athletic cup during the activity. The cup will increase the heat in the testicles—also a problem for fertility—but it's still safer than not wearing it.

Hold That Call

Landline phones may sound old-fashioned now, but they may be a safer bet when you're working toward fatherhood. Several studies have found a possible link between a man's cell phone usage and his fertility. One study, at the Cleveland Clinic in Ohio, found that the men who used their cell phones the most often had poorer quality sperm than the men who used them the least. Another study, at the University of Szeged in Hungary, found that men who had their phones on standby all day produced about a third fewer sperm than men who did not. Researchers warn that more studies are needed, but in the meantime, it wouldn't hurt to cut down on cell phone minutes for a while.

Keep That Laptop Away from Your Lap

Laptop computers are definitely not sperm-friendly technology. The machines generate heat and are positioned right on top of the genitals when they're perched on a lap. The male reproductive organs are outside the body to keep them cool, since a temperature lower than the body's core temperature is necessary for sperm production. When researchers asked men to hold a laptop computer on their laps, they found that the scrotal temperatures went up an average of nearly 5 degrees Fahrenheit (about 3 degrees Centigrade). Working with a laptop computer placed on a desk or table, however, is perfectly safe.

Keep Your Cool in Bed

Make your bedroom fertility-friendly by replacing waterbeds with regular mattresses, and electric blankets with the plain old cotton or wool kind. Researchers at the University of Pennsylvania and the University of Rochester have found that men who sleep on heated waterbeds are more likely to have fertility problems than men who sleep on regular beds. Electric blankets can also have this warming effect. So stick with an old-fashioned bed to produce your brand-new baby.

Fertility Facts

Boxers or Briefs?

And the winner is whichever one you prefer. It turns out that the age-old debate over whether boxers or briefs are better for conception doesn't really matter. Michael C. Darder, M.D., and Susan L. Treiser, M.D., Ph.D., board-certified reproductive endocrinologists and cofounders and codirectors of IVF New Jersey, recommend avoiding any tight-fitting nylon underwear that doesn't allow heat to escape from the groin area. But briefs in cotton or other fabrics that let skin breathe are just fine. So regardless of whether you like boxers or briefs, or if you prefer to "go commando," just remember to keep the scrotal temperature low.

The More,
The Better

While in theory it takes just one sperm to fertilize an egg, you actually need millions more for conception. While there's no magic number when it comes to sperm counts, doctors consider 20 million or more sperm per milliliter of ejaculation a normal number. In a typical ejaculation (about a teaspoon), 250 million sperm are released. According to Steven M. Schrader, Ph.D., leader of the reproductive health assessment team of the U.S. government's National Institute for Occupational Safety and Health, a low sperm count isn't the end of the world. It just means conception will take longer. And the number of sperm isn't the only measure of reproductive success. Male fertility is also dependent on sperm morphology (shape) and sperm motility (movement).

Danger in the Medicine Cabinet

Prescription medications and over-the-counter herbal remedies may have an effect on male fertility. That's why it's important to check your medicine cabinet early in the "trying" game. Antidepressant medication like Prozac, Paxil, and Zoloft can alter libido and the ability to get an erection or ejaculate. These drugs may also damage sperm and make them unable to fertilize an egg. Antihypertensives, which are potassium-sparing diuretics used to treat high blood pressure by ridding the body of excess water and salt, can impact male fertility by diminishing the sperm's ability to fertilize an egg. Ulcer medications can cause impotence in 40 percent of men, and sulfasalazine (which is used to treat inflammatory bowel diseases, such as Crohn's) can also reduce sperm counts. Even herbal remedies like echinacea, ginkgo biloba, and St. John's wort may hamper fertility. Check with your doctor to make sure anything you take is fertility-friendly before you start trying.

Just for Men

Snip, Tuck, Reverse?

Sometimes in life, things change. And that may be why approximately 1 percent of men who have had a vasectomy will eventually want a reversal so they can become fathers again (or for the first time). The good news is that most vasectomies can be successfully reversed with microsurgery, which succeeds about 90 percent of the time according to Sherman J. Silber, M.D., head of The Infertility Center of Saint Louis, Missouri. And when it doesn't, high-tech fertility treatments such as intracytoplasmic sperm injection, or ICSI, in which a single sperm is recovered and then inserted directly into an egg, can help.

Fertility Facts

Job Satisfaction

Exposure to certain toxins can threaten fertility, and employers are required to provide their workers with details about the types of materials they're working with. But according to Steven M. Schrader, Ph.D., team leader of the reproductive health assessment team at the National Institute for Occupational Safety and Health, it can be tough getting some employers to acknowledge the importance of reproductive health issues. He adds, "Some tend to say things like, 'Look at Joe over there. He's got five kids, so the situation can't be all that bad.'" If you're concerned about potential problems, do some research on your own and then talk with your employer.

HIV and Fatherhood

Being HIV-positive no longer means that fatherhood is forbidden. According to Michael C. Darder, M.D., and Susan L. Treiser, M.D., Ph.D., board-certified reproductive endocrinologists and cofounders and codirectors of IVF New Jersey, men with HIV can impregnate a woman relatively safely through sperm washing and the ICSI procedure. With sperm washing, sperm cells are separated from the rest of the ejaculatory fluid in the laboratory; the procedure gets rid of toxins (such as the HIV virus), dead sperm cells, and other chemicals that could impair fertilization. A single HIV-free sperm cell is then injected into the egg.

Clear the Air

Air pollution may be bad for more than the lungs. According to one recent study, the more smog in the air, the lower the sperm count of the men who breathe it. Researchers at the Keck School of Medicine of University of Southern California in Los Angeles compared men's sperm counts with the ozone levels where they lived. They found that the higher the ozone level, the lower the sperm count. Men who live in rural areas with lots of fresh air have no worries. But those who live in an urban area with frequently bad air quality might want to jog on an indoor track or install air filters at home.

Lose or Gain Weight If You Need To

A woman's weight can affect her chances of getting pregnant (see page 159). But so can a man's. Men who are either underweight or overweight can have fertility problems as a result. Researchers studied 1,500 Danish men and found that having a BMI of less than 20, or greater than 25, tended to lower sperm count and concentration. So stand on that scale, take a look in the mirror, and do the math to calculate your BMI (see page 171). Then do what you need to do to get yourself into fighting—and fertile—form.

Under Pressure

Stress affects more than just mental and physical well-being. It can also affect a man's sperm and lead to fertility problems. Marc Goldstein, M.D., director of the Center for Male Reproductive Medicine and Microsurgery at Weill Medical College of Cornell University in New York City, points out that stress has been shown to both lower sperm volume and raise the percentage of abnormal sperm. He advises men to learn how to manage stress through exercise or meditation. If all else fails, seek professional help.

Stay Away
From Steroids

Men may take anabolic steroids (such as testosterone) to look more macho and muscled, but the results may be anything but manly. Too much testosterone sometimes can "feminize" men, shrinking testicles and cutting sperm count and quality. It may take up to six months for fertility to return after discontinuing use. According to Machelle Seibel, M.D., professor of obstetrics and gynecology at the University of Massachusetts Medical School in Worcester, anabolic steroids can even sometimes make men permanently sterile.

Fertility Facts

Equal Opportunity Fertility Threats

Many people assume that trouble getting pregnant is usually a woman's problem, when in fact the fertility problem is just as often from the male side. It's estimated that in about 30 percent of infertility cases, the male is solely responsible for the problem, according to Larry I. Lipshultz, M.D., chief of the division of male reproductive medicine and surgery at Baylor College of Medicine in Houston, Texas. (Another 30 percent comes from the woman, and the remainder are the result of both male and female factors, or are undiagnosed and unexplained.) Experts recommend early screening for infertility problems, especially in men over 40, who should think about consulting a doctor after six months if conception hasn't happened. Younger men can wait up to a year, depending on their doctor's recommendations. The good news is 70 percent of male infertility cases are treatable.

Plumbing Problems

Varicoceles—varicose veins in the scrotum—are the leading cause of male fertility problems. With the average male producing 50,000 to 60,000 sperm per minute, or about 1,000 per second, problems can arise when one or more veins in a scrotum sac become enlarged, usually because of a faulty valve. Varicoceles occur in 35 to 40 percent of men who are screened for infertility. Doctors aren't sure how these abnormal veins impair fertility, but there are several theories. One is that the extra blood increases the internal temperature of the testes, which affects sperm quality and production. Another suggests that men with varicoceles experience a drop in testosterone levels. Still another theory posits that poor drainage in the testicles leaves the sperm exposed to toxins. Once detected, varicoceles can be surgically repaired. The surgery is done on an outpatient basis, and approximately 50 to 60 percent of men who have the surgery will be able to get their partners pregnant within two years.

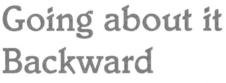

Going about it Backward

Retrograde ejaculation occurs in less than 1 percent of men. It's not a life-threatening condition; in fact, it's not really a problem until you're trying to conceive. In a normal ejaculation, semen flows out of the body to where it can potentially fertilize an egg. But in men with retrograde ejaculation, the semen flows backward into the bladder, where eventually it passes out of the body with urine. In fact, one telltale sign of the condition is urine that's cloudy (with semen) after orgasm. Doctors can help men with this condition to become fathers by collecting a urine sample after orgasm, washing it in the lab to separate out the sperm, and then using the sperm for an intrauterine insemination (IUI).

Chapter

9

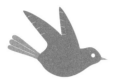

Sex Ed for Babymaking

You can learn everything there is to know about ovulation time and fertile dates and luteal phases and all that scientific stuff, but when it comes right down to it, good old-fashioned sex is the down-and-dirty, nitty-gritty way that most babies are made (we'll get into what to do when sex doesn't work in the next chapter). It doesn't matter if you like your sex plain, fancy, adventurous, fast, or slow. When it comes to making a baby, timing is the most important factor, but not the only one. For instance, bet you didn't know that the kind of foreplay you enjoy can make a difference in whether or not you conceive. Wonder whether a female orgasm makes a difference? Here's a quick guide to everything they didn't teach you in school about how to make a baby the old-fashioned way.

Assume the Position

No, you don't have to have sex in the missionary position night after night to conceive. In fact, you should choose positions that you like so you keep your interest strong while you're trying. Some women worry that if they're on top, gravity will work against conception. But sperm are speedy little swimmers who can make their way into the fallopian tubes in seconds. John R. Sussman, M.D., assistant clinical professor of obstetrics and gynecology at the University of Connecticut School of Medicine in Farmington, recommends that couples try any position that allows ejaculation deep in the vagina, which can happen in almost any position. And if missionary is your favorite position, there's no harm in sticking with it. And no, you don't need to lie in bed with your legs up in the air after sex.

More Is Not Necessarily Better

You may start your make-a-baby project so enthusiastically that you want to make love with your partner every day, or even more. Control yourself. More is not better when it comes to babymaking sex. Every man is different in terms of how fast his sperm count rebounds after ejaculation, but ejaculating too often can lower the numbers. Men may think they can "produce" every night, or several times a night! But the ability to ejaculate and the ability to ejaculate high-quality sperm are two different things. Most fertility doctors recommend that couples have intercourse every other day when they're trying to conceive. That schedule helps ensure that sperm will be potent and present during a woman's most fertile period.

Sex Ed for Babymaking

Oral Arguments

Foreplay is great before engaging in the main event, but you may want to hold off on oral sex while you're trying to get pregnant. According to a study at the Queen's University in Belfast, Ireland, saliva can significantly slow down a sperm's mobility by 50 percent in the first 5 minutes of intercourse and then by 95 percent within 15 minutes. So, at least while you're trying, stick with kisses on top only!

Fertility Facts

Practice a Different Kind of Safe Sex

Lubricants can help make intercourse more pleasurable, but if you're trying to conceive, experts recommend avoiding oil-based lubricants for now. According to Mark P. Leondires, M.D., a reproductive endocrinologist with Reproductive Medicine Associates of Connecticut in Norwalk, "oil-based lubricants or any product containing scents or inorganic materials are likely to kill sperm." Lubes can also affect sperm mobility, slowing down the swimmers. There are a few natural alternatives that are safe and effective. These include mineral oil, vegetable oil, corn oil, olive oil, or egg whites. But perhaps your best choice is to engage in such wonderful foreplay that you produce plenty of natural lubrication on your own, or look for lubricants that specifically advertise themselves as "sperm-friendly."

Sex Ed for Babymaking

The Ovulation Imperative

Timing is everything when it comes to conception. That's why experts recommend that every woman who is trying to get pregnant know her most fertile days, and then time sexual intercourse to take advantage of it. Knowing when you ovulate is important, but women are actually most fertile several days before. Once the egg is released, it starts to disintegrate fairly quickly if no sperm are present to fertilize it. But sperm can survive in the female reproductive tract for several days, so having sperm already waiting for a newly released egg is the best way to get pregnant.

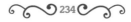

Even Regular Cycles Can Be Irregular

Keep in mind that even women with the most regular cycles can experience irregularity in ovulation. According to a study done at the National Institutes of Environmental Health Sciences, more than 70 percent of normal women were in their fertile window before day 10 or after day 17. So if a few months go by without success, you may want to try an ovulation predictor kit to double-check your most fertile period.

Boys to the Left

Some people want a boy, some people want a girl, but most just want a healthy baby. Still, sex selection is nothing new; it dates all the way back to the days of ancient Greece. The Greeks believed that if men had sex while on their right side a boy would result. In eighteenth-century France, it was believed that if men tied off their left testicle the couple would be blessed with a boy. Today, the only sure (or nearly sure) way to choose your baby's sex is by using preimplantation genetic diagnosis (PGD), which can actually check an embryo's sex before implantation and IVF. But this method, while nearly 100 percent certain, is used mostly for couples concerned about passing along sex-linked genetic diseases or conditions.

Fertility Facts

Is It Getting Hot in Here?

Contrary to popular belief, basal body temperature (BBT) monitoring isn't the ideal way to time intercourse for conception. That's because your fertility is highest during the two days prior to ovulation and on the day itself. But BBT changes 12 to 24 hours *after* ovulation. Since the egg lives only one day, by the time your BBT indicates you're ovulating, you've only got a tiny fertile window in which to conceive. The method, however, can help identify a condition known as luteal phase defect, in which your body produces insufficient levels of progesterone, the hormone crucial for implantation.

Sex Ed for Babymaking

Exercise for Better Sex and Better Pregnancy

You don't even have to get off the couch to do one exercise that can help your sex life now, and your pregnancy later: Kegels. This exercise targets the pelvic floor muscles that are important for general pelvic health and sexual response. First, you can find where these muscles are by trying to stop the flow of urine next time you use the bathroom. The muscles you contract are the ones you're targeting. Next, practice tightening these muscles for a count of 4 and then relaxing them, repeating the exercise 10 to 20 times a day. You'll feel a difference in just a couple of months.

The Big O
and Pregnancy

While men certainly need an orgasm for babymaking, women don't need the big finish to conceive. In theory, an orgasm could help a woman get pregnant, but experts agree it's not necessary. When you have an orgasm, your uterus contracts, causing a vacuum effect. Theoretically, that "sucking effect" could help boost the sperm into the uterus. But as medical experts including John R. Sussman, M.D., assistant clinical professor of obstetrics and gynecology at the University of Connecticut School of Medicine in Farmington, point out, there isn't any scientific evidence that shows orgasms help. As far as conceiving goes, focus on the timing of intercourse first, and then enjoy the extra benefit of an orgasm if it happens.

Sex Ed for Babymaking

The Crackpot Theory of Swimming Pool Pregnancies

It sounds like one of those unsolved old wives' tale mysteries about getting pregnant circulated for decades. In the early 1900s there was a theory that claimed women could become pregnant by swimming in the same swimming pool as men. People rationalized that spermatozoa in the water could swim from one person to another and voilà! Popular newspaper columnist Ann Landers nipped this crackpot theory in the bud when she devoted an entire column to preposterous pregnancy legends.

Don't Worry
If It Leaks

Don't worry if the sperm leaks out after sex. The fluid that carries the sperm is thick and gummy during ejaculation and then liquefies 30 to 60 minutes later. "Each ejaculation is about 2 or 3 cubic centimeters, and each cc has 20 to 80 million sperm in it," explains Mary Jane Minkin, M.D., clinical professor of obstetrics and gynecology at Yale University School of Medicine in New Haven, Connecticut. "So if a few guys escape, it's no big deal."

Sex Ed for Babymaking

Loosen Up
Your Foreplay

Massaging each other is a great way to get in the mood. It can help you relax and can even be beneficial for your relationship, especially if you aren't conceiving as quickly as you'd like. Research has found that massage decreases levels of the stress hormone cortisol, and increases levels of the brain chemicals serotonin and dopamine, both of which are associated with experiencing pleasure. When conception sex is starting to become a chore, preceding your encounter with a sensuous couples' massage can get you relaxed and back in the mood.

Fertility Facts

Afternoon Delight

The Starland Vocal Band may have been on to something with their sexually suggestive song "Afternoon Delight" in 1976. The time of day couples have sex may play a role in conception. Journalist Lynne Lamberg, coauthor of the book *The Body Clock Guide to Better Health* (Henry Holt and Co., 2001), cites an Italian study at the University of Modena, which found men produce more and faster sperm in the afternoon. Who needs an excuse to cut out of work early for a little romantic rendezvous between the sheets?

Sex Ed for Babymaking

Newlywed Bliss

Ever wondered why you see newlyweds glowing and flushed all the time? Experts say newlyweds often have sex two to three times a week. That's also the recommended sex schedule for couples trying to conceive in order to optimize sperm numbers and conception rates. Philip E. Chenette, M.D., a reproductive endocrinologist at Pacific Fertility Center in San Francisco, California, says, "One of the biggest mistakes patients [trying to conceive] make is losing sight of their relationship." So think back to those newlywed days and remember that Mother Nature always knows best.

Fertility Facts

Keep It Steamy

It's tough to make a baby the old-fashioned way if you stop having sex, and that's what can happen to some couples when months of "trying" don't result in a pregnancy. What starts out as a sexy, fun project—finally it's OK to have unprotected sex!—can quickly become a chore and a bore. Take some tips from the sex experts to keep it steamy so you don't lose interest in this important collaboration. For instance, try abstaining from sex all month except during your fertile period; you'll definitely be in the mood when it's time! Book a night in a hotel to coincide with your next fertile phase. Try new positions, new lingerie, and even porn movies: anything that will keep things from getting boring.

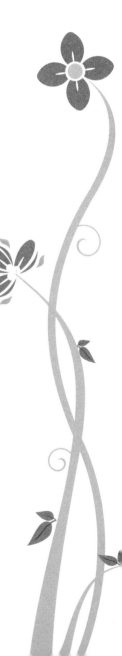

Sex Ed for Babymaking

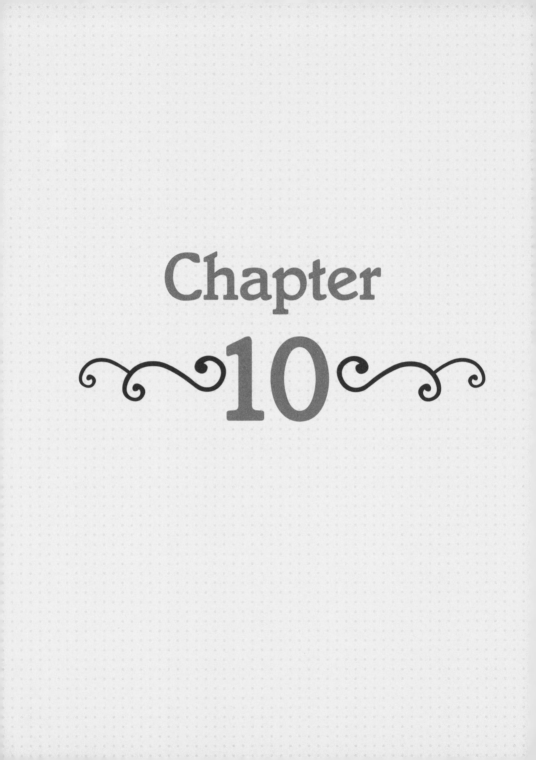

Chapter
10

Assisted Reproduction and Other Medical Help

You've had your checkup, taken your vitamins, watched your weight, and had lots and lots of sex. But you're still not pregnant. Now what? It might be time to ask for some help from modern medicine. Fortunately, the medical arsenal of infertility treatments is big and growing bigger. Medication, surgical techniques, and high-tech fertility procedures like IVF (in vitro fertilization) mean that nearly everyone who wants to be a biological parent can be. In fact, fertility treatments are becoming so successful that many doctors don't consider their patients infertile, but subfertile, meaning they'll be able to become pregnant with help. So if you're among the millions who need that help, here's what might be in store.

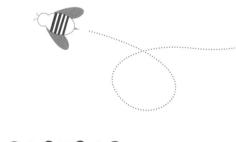

The One-Year Rule

If you're under 35 and you haven't conceived after one year of trying, you should seek medical help. A proper fertility workup should begin with a complete physical for woman and man, as well as thorough reviews of both partners' medical and sexual histories. If she hasn't already been doing it, the woman should start tracking her ovulation, either with a home kit or a home monitoring device provided by her doctor, by tracking her BBT, or by having a blood progesterone test at the doctor's office.

His and Hers Tests

A basic fertility workup for men and women includes some standard tests. For men, the first test is always to give a sperm sample; a lab analysis will measure the amount (sperm count), shape and appearance (morphology), and movement (motility). If the sperm doesn't test normal, further tests will try to determine why. For women, tests may include a hysterosalpingogram—an X-ray of the fallopian tubes and uterus—to see if the tubes are blocked by scar tissue, preventing the egg from being fertilized.

Assisted Reproduction and Other Medical Help

The Six-Month Shortcut

Women 35 and older don't have the luxury of time. Those who haven't become pregnant after six months of trying should see a fertility specialist, and not wait a year. In addition to the basic fertility workup, the doctor should do a blood test on day 3 of your cycle to check your ovarian reserve, the supply of healthy eggs left in your ovaries. The test should measure estradiol, follicle stimulating hormone (FSH), luteinizing hormone (LH, which triggers ovulation), and inhibin B, a hormone that controls FSH secretion. If the ovaries are healthy, FSH will be low and inhibin B high.

Fertility Facts

Ready, eSET, Go!

The debate over how many embryos to implant for in vitro fertilization (IVF) continues. On the one hand, most doctors still believe that the more embryos implanted, the greater the chance for success. On the other hand, implanting multiple embryos raises the risk of multiple births—twins, triplets, and even higher. And pregnancies of multiples are riskier, with greater dangers for the mother and the babies (who are more likely to be born prematurely). That's why many experts are now calling for clinics to use elective Single Embryo Transfer—eSET. Their reasoning is that with new and better ways to evaluate embryos, doctors can better predict which embryos are most likely to lead to a successful pregnancy. Some European countries, including Iceland, Finland, and Sweden, have already adopted eSET, and others are following suit. In the United States, the American Society for Reproductive Medicine is recommending that doctors consider eSET in women under 35. Of course, individual cases require individual decisions. Women undergoing IVF should discuss their situation with their doctor to determine the number that's right for them.

Assisted Reproduction and Other Medical Help

It Can Be Harder the Second Time

Most couples assume that once they've already had a child together, having another won't be difficult. Yet 3 million people in America experience secondary infertility, which is defined as the inability to conceive a baby or carry a pregnancy to term after the birth of one or more children. In fact, experts say secondary infertility is actually more common than primary infertility. Sometimes the only difference is the passage of time. A couple that was in their early thirties for the birth of their first child may be in their late thirties by the time they try again. And that difference in age—and women's fertility—can make it harder the second time.

Different Name, Same Causes

Just as with primary infertility, secondary infertility can be the result of a myriad of causes, and can originate with the man or the woman or both. According to Daniel F. Rychlik, M.D., a reproductive endocrinologist specializing in infertility and associate medical director of the Fertility Treatment Center in Scottsdale and Tempe, Arizona, the most common causes in women involve ovulation disorders, early menopause, pelvic adhesions, inflammation or infection, damage or blockage of the fallopian tubes, uterine fibroids or polyps, and endometriosis. Men can experience low or no sperm count, impaired mobility, ejaculation problems, or poor-quality sperm. Fortunately, secondary infertility can usually be quickly diagnosed and treated.

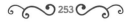

Assisted Reproduction and Other Medical Help

Less Stress, More IVF Success

How much stress a woman is exposed to and how she experiences it may affect her chance of IVF success. In 2004, a study published in the medical journal *Fertility and Sterility* showed a connection between the stress of receiving fertility treatments and the success or failure of those treatments. Translation: Less-stressed patients had higher success rates. Hillary Klonoff-Cohen, Ph.D., a professor in the department of family and preventive medicine at the University of California, San Diego, found that among the 151 patients in her study, the women who were extremely concerned about the fertility procedures (the expense, anesthetic, pain, and success) were three times less likely to get pregnant and eleven times less likely to carry a pregnancy to term. Since stress is pretty much unavoidable for couples undergoing fertility treatments, counseling is recommended if the stress is disruptive to daily life or may be affecting the success of treatment.

Fertility Facts

Just the Facts, Ma'am

Before a couple decides to visit a fertility specialist, they should do some homework. Fertility clinics will often inundate potential patients with information about their success rates, and the maze of information can be overwhelming. The U.S. Centers for Disease Control and Prevention mandates that all IVF clinics report their success rates annually, and according to Eric S. Surrey, M.D., past president of the Society for Assisted Reproductive Technology and medical director at the Colorado Center for Reproductive Medicine in Englewood, over 90 percent of them do. An individual clinic's statistics can be found online at www.cdc.gov/ART/.

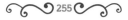

Making Sense of the Numbers

The statistics that a fertility clinic provides will list how many patients have been treated, and in what age groups. Look for the live-birth rate, suggests Owen K. Davis, M.D., associate director of IVF at The Center for Reproductive Medicine and Infertility, and chief of the division of gynecology at the Weill Medical College of Cornell University in New York City. Check how many women got pregnant, and then compare that number to how many took home a baby. Under age 35, the live-birth rate at the top clinics nationwide is 50 percent or higher. At age 40, the most successful programs have a live-birth rate in the high 20 to 30 percent range. Most important of all, look for the statistics that most closely match your age and situation.

Another Reason to Quit

Here's yet another reason to stamp out the cancer sticks: quitting smoking not only improves natural fertility, it also ups your chances of conceiving with IVF, says Richard E. Leach, M.D., director of the division of reproductive endocrinology and infertility at the University of Illinois in Chicago. Dr. Leach points out that people who smoke during IVF treatments cut their chances of getting pregnant in half. Experts say that smoking may affect the lining of the uterus or the outer layer of the egg. But quitting improves the odds of getting pregnant. According to one study, stopping smoking for at least two months prior to treatment can significantly increase the likelihood of conception. Scientists have also found that smoking makes a woman reproductively 10 years older—meaning that a 30-year-old smoker has the same chance of getting pregnant with IVF as a 40-year-old nonsmoker.

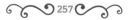

History Isn't Destiny

There's hope for couples with a history of genetic diseases (such as muscular dystrophy or Huntington's disease) who want to make sure they don't pass on those conditions to their offspring. Doctors can use preimplantation genetic diagnosis (PGD) with IVF to look at a three-day-old embryo and select only the embryos free of that disease to implant. According to Michael C. Darder, M.D., and Susan L. Treiser, M.D., Ph.D., board-certified reproductive endocrinologists and cofounders and codirectors of IVF New Jersey, physicians can only study a small percentage of an embryo's chromosomes, so doctors can't really determine if an embryo is completely genetically healthy or not. For this reason, PGD is most often recommended for couples who need to be screened for a specific genetic problem.

Fertility Facts

When Sperm Attack

Strangely enough, it's actually possible for a woman to be allergic to her partner's sperm. Sperm antibodies occur in approximately 5 percent of couples seeking fertility treatments, and these antibodies can attack the sperm, immobilizing them or making them incapable of fertilizing an egg. In this case, a woman's body is reacting to the sperm as it would to a foreign invader. Men can also become allergic to their own sperm, producing antibodies against it, although this condition only occurs when the testicles have been injured, or a man has had testicular surgery. In either case, doctors can use intrauterine inseminations (IUIs) or IVF treatments to help counteract the antibodies and achieve pregnancy.

Assisted Reproduction and Other Medical Help

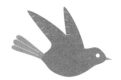

It Only Takes One

There's new hope for men suffering from fertility challenges. A technique called intracytoplasmic sperm injection (ICSI) can take a single sperm cell and inject it directly into an egg to help spur fertilization. With this technique, even men with extremely low sperm counts can be helped to become fathers. According to Marc Goldstein, M.D., director of the Center for Male Reproductive Medicine and Microsurgery at the Weill Medical College of Cornell University in New York City, 60 percent of men with zero sperm counts and a history of undescended testes see success with ICSI.

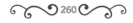

Generous Donations

Sperm banks and donor sperm have been around for decades. But with new developments like intracytoplasmic sperm injection (ICSI), which inserts a single sperm into an egg cell, fewer and fewer men are incapable of becoming biological fathers. That means the use of donor sperm is waning among couples (although still popular with single women who want to become mothers). Instead, the use of donor eggs is rising, as more women are waiting until later in life to become mothers. When older women can't get pregnant using their own eggs, donor eggs from younger women can often help. The newest fertility donations, though, are embryo donations: couples who have leftover embryos after IVF can opt to donate them to infertile couples.

Assisted Reproduction and Other Medical Help

Tipping the Scales

Research shows that being overweight (that's defined as having a BMI of at least 25) can make it tougher for a woman to get pregnant. But carrying around extra pounds can also hamper the success of fertility treatments. The effect is pronounced enough that many fertility clinics now set BMI limits for women—usually 35, sometimes 40—before accepting them as patients. Randy S. Morris, M.D., a reproductive endocrinologist and medical director of IVF1 in Chicago and ·Naperville, Illinois, says his center has seen the percentage of obese women seeking fertility treatments climb from 9 to 39 percent over a three-year period. Clinics say the BMI limits are necessary because IVF is considered less safe and less likely to be successful in severely overweight women.

Fertility Facts

Shopping for Eggs

More than 11 percent of high-tech fertility treatments, such as IVF, now involve donor eggs. In fact, as of 2002 when the most recent government numbers were published, over 13,000 IVF attempts were performed using donor eggs. With an average live birth per transfer rate of 50 percent, that means more than 6,000 babies are born each year as a result of their mothers using another woman's eggs. The biggest determining factor in whether or not a woman uses donor eggs is her age. Few women younger than age 39 use donor eggs, but the use increases sharply among women age 40 and above. After age 45, more than three-quarters of all assisted reproductive technology cycles use donor eggs.

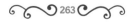

Womb for Rent

Surrogates aren't what they used to be. In traditional surrogacy, a woman was inseminated with a man's sperm (or the embryo was created in vitro—in the lab) and then she carried the pregnancy to term. So the surrogate was the biological mother of the child she carried. This arrangement could be difficult, both legally and personally, since the surrogate had a strong biological and physical connection to the child she bore. Now surrogates are much more likely to be "gestational carriers," meaning that they become pregnant with an embryo created with another woman's egg—either an egg from the woman who will be the child's mother, or an egg donor.

Fertility Facts

Fresh Eggs

Here's another reason to have age on your side when trying to have a baby. The younger a woman is when she tries assisted reproductive technology (or ART, which includes fertility procedures where sperm and egg are handled in a laboratory), the more likely she is to have a baby using her own eggs. The U.S. Centers for Disease Control and Prevention released statistics in 2002 showing that there's a decidedly higher rate of ART success for women under age 35. Thirty-seven percent of women under age 35 were able to deliver babies using non-donor ART procedures. By age 35 to 37, that rate dropped to 31 percent. From age 38 to 40 the rate was 21 percent and from age 41 to 42 there was only an 11 percent success rate. After age 42, only 4 percent of women were able to become pregnant and deliver a child using their own eggs.

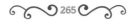

Assisted Reproduction and Other Medical Help

Boys Are
Worth the Wait

With natural conception, the chance of having a boy is approximately 50 percent. But the same isn't necessarily true with IVF. Researchers at the Mount Sinai School of Medicine and Reproductive Medicine Associates in New York City analyzed data from their fertility center and found that the timing of embryo transfer affected the sex ratio of the resulting births. Specifically, the researchers found that when the embryos were transferred on the third day after harvesting and culturing, the sex ratio was approximately the same as that with natural conception (about 51 percent male and 49 percent female). But when day 5 embryos—called blastocysts—were transferred, the sex ratio was seriously skewed. Almost 58 percent of babies born as a result of these transfers were male. And when the researchers analyzed only singleton births, the ratio was 64 percent male to 36 percent female. More research is needed to figure out the reason for this phenomenon, but couples who care about the sex of their child can keep this information in mind when planning IVF cycles.

Fertility Facts

Light Up Your IVF

Light may boost the fertility quotient of women undergoing IVF. Some studies suggest that procedures done in the summer months, when there is more daylight, have a greater percent of success than those done at times of the year with less light—one study indicated a 4 percent increase in success rates. That may be because light affects the pineal gland, which produces melatonin, a hormone that may enhance ovulation. A study published in 2006 in the journal *Human Fertility* showed that IVF rates spike in June, July, and August (even though sperm counts may decrease then due to the higher temperatures).

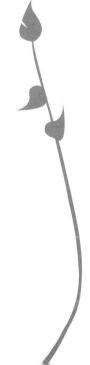

Assisted Reproduction and Other Medical Help

Light Up Your IVF Clinic

A researcher in Hawaii has found that the kind of lighting used in fertility clinics can affect whether the embryos successfully develop into babies. Ryuzo Yanagimachi, Ph.D., a retired professor of anatomy and reproductive biology at the University of Hawai'i at Manoa, exposed mice embryos to various kinds of lighting and found that warm-white light was the least damaging, while sunlight and cool-white fluorescent lights (the kind in most offices) caused the most damage to the embryos, even when the exposure was limited to a few minutes. Yanagimachi believes that human embryos may be similarly affected by light.

Fertility Facts

Send in the Clowns

Fertility treatments may not seem like something to laugh about, but smiling and giggling may be one of the best things you can do during IVF. Researchers at the Assaf Harofeh Medical Center in Israel studied women who were undergoing embryo transfers—the part of IVF when the embryos are placed in the womb. Half of the women were entertained by a clown for up to 15 minutes as they rested in bed after the treatment. Of the 93 women in the clowning group, 33 became pregnant. But only 18 of the control group became pregnant. Based on this and other studies, many experts now believe that helping women relax is one key to increasing IVF conception rates.

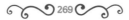

A Silver Lining, Sort Of

Women who have infertility problems because of an ovulation disorder may have a lower risk of breast cancer than women who have no difficulty conceiving. That small comfort comes from a data analysis of the over 116,000 women enrolled in the Harvard *Nurses' Health Study II*. Overall, the women who had ovulatory disorders had a 25 percent lower likelihood of developing breast cancer. Perhaps even more surprising, the risk was lowest in the women who had taken fertility drugs to induce ovulation.

Please Explain

Roughly 15 percent of all infertility is unexplained, meaning that doctors are unable to find the reason why conception isn't occurring. It may be that it just takes some couples longer to get pregnant, and conception would occur after the one-year "cutoff" for an infertility diagnosis has passed. Or there may be some fertility problems so subtle that science still can't detect them. But just because infertility is unexplained doesn't mean it can't be overcome. For younger couples, patience may be all that's needed. For those who are older, or just don't want to wait, fertility treatments can often help.

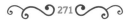

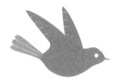

Birth Control For Babies?

You might think that birth control pills would be the last thing you'd take when you're trying to have a baby, but oral contraceptives have a role in fertility treatments. A standard round of IVF starts with suppressing a woman's normal menstrual cycle using birth control pills and other drugs to stop the production of the hormones FSH and LH. This allows the doctor to control the timing of the cycle.

The Test Can Be the Cure

One of the first tests a woman may have as part of a fertility workup is the hysterosalpingogram, an X-ray of the uterus and surrounding area to see if the fallopian tubes are blocked and whether there are uterine abnormalities. A dye is injected through a catheter, and then the X-ray photos can show whether or not the dye was able to pass through the tubes. According to some research, the test itself may be the cure. Studies have found that when this "tubal flushing" is done with an oil-soluble rather than water-soluble media, pregnancy rates rise without any further treatment. It may be that simply passing the fluid through the tubes is enough to remove some blockages and clear a pathway for sperm and egg to meet.

Assisted Reproduction and Other Medical Help

Two Tests to Skip

When you're trying to figure out why you're not conceiving, you'll obviously be subjected to a lot of tests as your doctors search for a diagnosis. But there are two tests, still sometimes recommended, that experts believe to be a waste of time and money. One test, an endometrial biopsy, checks for luteal defects—problems with the menstrual cycle between ovulation and menstruation. The other test is called a postcoital test—a check of cervical mucus, sperm, and the interaction between the two, taken right after sexual intercourse. According to the American Society for Reproductive Medicine, neither of these tests has been shown to improve pregnancy rates.

Fertility Facts

Drug of Choice

There's one medication that nearly every woman experiencing ovulatory fertility problems will take at some point: clomiphene citrate (brand names in the United States include Clomid and Serophene). The effect of this drug is like "hitting the reset button on a woman's cycle," says William D. Schlaff, M.D., professor of obstetrics and gynecology and chief of reproductive endocrinology at the University of Colorado Health Sciences Center in Denver. This pill works by tricking the body into thinking it's low in estrogen, so that more is produced. An estimated half to two-thirds of all couples with fertility challenges will be treated with clomiphene at some point. And many, many of them will get pregnant without having to go on to more expensive and high-tech treatments.

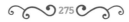

Take Two and Call When You're Pregnant

The old doctors' cliché—"Take two aspirin and call me in the morning"—might become a new treatment for miscarriage. A study at the Sheba Medical Center in Israel found that for women who had suffered recurrent miscarriages with no known cause, treatment with aspirin or other blood thinners seemed to improve the chance of a successful pregnancy. Blood clots are believed to be one possible cause of recurrent miscarriages.

One in One Hundred

We've come a long way. Since Louise Brown, the world's first "test tube baby" was born in Britain in 1978, more than 3 million children worldwide have been born as a result of IVF. Today assisted reproductive technology, including IVF, accounts for a bit more than 1 percent of all U.S. births.

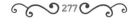

Hypnotize Yourself Pregnant

Researchers from Soroka University Medical Center in Israel have found that women who are hypnotized before the embryo transfer stage of an IVF may be more likely to get pregnant. One possible explanation is that the hypnosis helps keep the uterus relaxed and more receptive to the embryo. Hypnotherapy is also sometimes used as part of fertility treatment to help women conceive, but evidence of its success is anecdotal. Still, hypnosis does seem to work as a form of stress reduction, so if it's part of fertility relaxation therapy, it may help and almost certainly can't hurt.

Fertility Facts

IVF, Naturally?

For some women, the large doses of hormones and other fertility drugs used in IVF may be hazardous. For instance, women who've been treated for certain types of cancer may worry that the hormones will cause the cancer to recur or grow. In this case, doctors can try so-called natural IVF. In natural IVF, no fertility drugs are involved. Doctors wait for a woman's natural ovulation, and then harvest the single ripened egg for fertilization and implantation. In fact, this is how IVF was performed decades ago, when the procedure was still new. Now, most IVF involves using powerful drugs to stimulate the ovaries to ripen many eggs, increasing the odds of pregnancy success. But for women, especially younger women, who are willing to accept the trade-off of a lower success rate in exchange for avoiding fertility drugs, natural IVF is one option to consider.

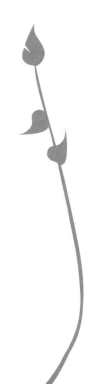

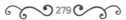

Fewer Drugs, Not Fewer Babies

Between regular IVF and natural IVF (which uses no fertility drugs) there is a third option, called minimal-stimulation IVF. Since the trend in IVF is to implant as few embryos as possible (and ideally just a single embryo, to avoid the risk of a multiple pregnancy), some doctors are questioning whether it's still necessary to stimulate a woman's ovaries with powerful hormones that can help produce large numbers of eggs but come with large side effects, too. The New Hope Fertility Center in New York City is pioneering a procedure called minimal-stimulation IVF (also called MS-IVF or Mini-IVF) that relies only on the oral drug clomiphene citrate, and involves no injections at all. Instead of suppressing a woman's natural cycle, the way most IVF procedures do, Mini-IVF uses a woman's own cycle, with the result being ovulation induction with fewer drugs.

Freezing Fertility

Although egg freezing is still a relatively new procedure (and some consider it still experimental), more and more women are considering it if they reach their thirties and are still unattached or are immersed in a career and not ready for children. The hope is that by freezing their eggs when they're younger, they will be more likely to get pregnant when they're finally ready. In the past, egg freezing was so uncertain a prospect that it was generally only recommended for women undergoing cancer therapy who had few other options for preserving their fertility. Younger women who are tested and found to have a low ovarian reserve—meaning few viable eggs left in the ovaries—also have a medical reason to consider the procedure. But as the technique for freezing eggs becomes more refined and successful, even healthy women who are worried about aging eggs are opting to freeze some of their own as a kind of fertility insurance policy.

Coldest Record

How long can sperm be frozen and still create a healthy baby? At least 21 years, according to British scientists at St. Mary's Hospital for Women & Children in Manchester, England. Doctors there reported that in 2002 a healthy baby boy was born to a couple decades after the father had been treated for testicular cancer and frozen his sperm. Just 17 years old when he was diagnosed, the father had five vials of sperm frozen before he underwent surgery, radiation, and chemotherapy for his cancer, because doctors told him it would leave him sterile. Years later when the man was married and the couple wished to be parents, doctors defrosted the sperm and used intracytoplasmic sperm injection (ICSI), a procedure in which a single sperm is injected into an egg to fertilize it. The baby was the result of the couple's fourth IVF cycle.

Fertility Facts

The Low-Tech Majority

High-tech fertility treatments make the news so often that couples experiencing difficulty getting pregnant probably think that as soon as they visit the doctor they'll be put on the path to costly IVF. Not so. The majority of fertility problems—an estimated 85 to 90 percent—are still treated with conventional medical therapies such as medication or surgery.

Your Cycle Explained

A typical menstrual cycle is 28 days long, with menstruation occurring on day 1. Many women assume that ovulation occurs in the middle of their cycle, or they think that ovulation is always around day 14. In fact, ovulation doesn't occur 14 days after menstruation starts, but 14 days *before*. So a woman with a 32-day cycle would most likely ovulate around day 18, not 14. The entire fertile phase includes the day of ovulation, plus the few days preceding it (because sperm can live in the female reproductive tract for several days). Once ovulation has occurred, or immediately afterward, the fertile phase is over for that cycle.

One way to determine your own fertile period is to keep a record of your menstrual cycles for several months. Select your longest and shortest cycles, and subtract 18 to find the beginning of your fertile period. For instance, if your shortest cycle was 27 days long, and your longest was 32, your fertile period would start between days 9 and 12. Ovulation would occur between days 13 and 18. So your entire potentially fertile period would begin on day 9 and end on day 18.

This is still a very wide window of opportunity. You can narrow it further by charting your basal body temperature (your morning temperature before getting out of bed). For most women, it ranges from 96 to 98 degrees Fahrenheit. When your temperature rises slightly ($\frac{4}{10}$ to $\frac{8}{10}$ of a degree, measured with a special, extra-sensitive thermometer), it usually means you have ovulated within the past 12 to 24 hours. But you'll have to use this information as a guide to

Your Cycle Explained

conceiving for next month, because by the time you determine you're ovulating, the fertile window for the cycle has probably passed.

One more method of identifying your fertile period is to notice changes in your cervical mucus. The mucus ranges from dry (following menstruation) to sticky (approaching ovulation) to wet, stretchy, and semitransparent (during ovulation). Ovulation usually occurs from two days before to two days after the peak day of stretchy mucus.

While, as mentioned above, every woman's cycle varies slightly, here's a day-by-day account of what happens during an average 28-day cycle as the body prepares for a possible pregnancy.

Days 1 to 5 If you are not pregnant, old dead tissue lining the uterus sloughs off, and menstruation begins. Estrogen and progesterone levels are low. Body temperature is 96 to 98 degrees Fahrenheit.

Days 6 to 7 The hypothalamus, a brain structure that regulates the internal organs and controls the pituitary gland, secretes gonadotropin releasing hormone (GnRH). GnRH, in turn, tells the pituitary to release follicle stimulating hormone (FSH) and luteinizing hormone (LH), which cause the eggs, or follicles, in one of the ovaries to begin growing. As the eggs grow, they produce estrogen. Progesterone remains low. Cervical mucus is dry (through days 8 or 9).

Day 8 (may extend to day 12) Secretion of estrogen increases, which causes the lining of the uterus to become thicker and generate a richer supply of blood vessels, preparing it to receive a fertilized egg. FSH and LH levels decline.

Day 10 Mucus becomes wet with cloudy, sticky, or whitish or yellowish secretions.

Day 12 Mucus becomes clear, slippery, and stretchy, signaling ovulation is near. You are most likely to become pregnant during this period. (Sperm survive for two to five days after intercourse, which is why sex now can lead to pregnancy even though ovulation is still several days away.)

Day 13 Estrogen rises dramatically, which boosts LH. LH stimulates the synthesis of progesterone, which causes FSH to rise. Within 12 hours of ovulation, body temperature rises between $\frac{4}{10}$ and $\frac{8}{10}$ of a degree and, if pregnancy does not occur, remains high until the next menstrual period.

Day 14 Estrogen falls sharply and LH surges, which causes the ovary to release the egg—ovulation. The egg lives for about 12 to 24 hours.

Day 15 (may extend to day 24) The empty egg follicle—the corpus luteum—secretes increasing amounts of estrogen and progesterone to help prepare the uterus for a possible pregnancy. FSH and LH levels begin to drop.

Day 17 When your body temperature has stayed high for three days in a row, generally your fertile period is over.

Day 18 Cervical mucus becomes cloudy.

Days 21 to 22 Progesterone level peaks.

Your Cycle Explained

Day 25 The corpus luteum breaks apart. If the egg was not fertilized, progesterone begins to drop and cervical mucus is tacky. (If fertilization occurred, your progesterone level remains high.)

Day 27 Mucus is absent or dry.

Day 28 Estrogen level decreases and progesterone production rapidly drops. Mucus is thick. If you're not pregnant, your period will begin tomorrow.

Your Fertile Dictionary

You may sometimes feel that you need a medical degree to understand the biology of conception and the terminology of fertility. Most confusing of all are the many initials and acronyms that get easily tossed around by gynecologists and fertility specialists. Use our handy-dandy decoder, below, for help.

AH Assisted hatching
The zona pellucida, or outer covering, of the embryo is partially opened, to aid implantation.

ART Assisted reproductive technology
A phrase to describe any treatments that involve handling human eggs or embryos.

CASA Computer-assisted semen analysis
A technique to measure and study sperm motion when male infertility is suspected.

CCCT Clomiphene citrate challenge test

A blood test to measure FSH (see below) taken on days 3 and 10 of the menstrual cycle. Clomiphene citrate is given on days 5 through 9 to induce ovulation.

EEJ Electroejaculation

A procedure that involves electrically stimulating tissue near a man's prostate to cause ejaculation.

FSH Follicle stimulating hormone

A hormone produced by the pituitary gland (and sometimes given by injection). FSH stimulates the growth of the follicle surrounding an egg.

GIFT Gamete intrafallopian transfer

The placing of sperm and egg directly into the fallopian tube, where fertilization takes place.

GnRH Gonadotropin releasing hormone

A hormone secreted by the hypothalamus (an area of the brain that controls reproduction and other actions) that prompts the pituitary gland to release FSH and LH into the bloodstream.

hCG Human chorionic gonadotropin

A hormone produced by the placenta that is measured in common pregnancy tests. It may also be injected to stimulate ovulation and maturation of eggs.

Your Cycle Explained

HMG Human menopausal gonadotropin

A medication containing FSH and LH derived from the urine of postmenopausal women. HMG is used to stimulate the growth of multiple egg follicles.

HSG Hysterosalpingogram

An X-ray procedure to check if the fallopian tubes are open and whether there are uterine abnormalities.

ICSI Intracytoplasmic sperm injection

A procedure in which a single sperm is injected directly into an egg to help spur fertilization, used primarily with male infertility.

IUI Intrauterine insemination

A form of artificial insemination in which sperm that has been washed free of seminal fluid to increase the chance of fertilization is inserted directly into the uterus.

IVF In vitro fertilization

A procedure in which an egg and sperm are combined in the laboratory to facilitate fertilization. Resulting embryos are transferred to a woman's uterus.

LH Luteinizing hormone

Produced by the pituitary gland, this hormone normally causes a woman to ovulate and her eggs to mature.

MESA Microepididymal sperm aspiration

A procedure for collecting sperm from men whose reproductive ducts are blocked, usually as a result of a vasectomy or absence of vas deferens.

OHSS Ovarian hyperstimulation syndrome

A potentially life-threatening condition characterized by enlargement of the ovaries, fluid retention, and weight gain that may occur when the ovaries are overstimulated during assisted reproduction.

PGD Preimplantation genetic diagnosis

One or two cells are removed from an embryo and screened for genetic abnormalities.

PESA Percutaneous epididymal sperm aspiration

A procedure in which a needle is inserted into the gland that carries sperm from the testicle to the vas deferens in order to extract sperm for an IVF procedure.

TESE Testicular sperm extraction

Surgery to remove testicular tissue and collect living sperm for use in an IVF or ICSI procedure.

ZIFT Zygote intrafallopian transfer

A procedure similar to IVF in which an egg is fertilized in a laboratory dish and the zygote (the stage before cell division begins) is transferred to the fallopian tube.

Your Cycle Explained

Pre-Conception Checklist

Ready to get pregnant? Not so fast! Before you toss the contraceptives, take a few steps first to make sure your body—and your partner's—is ready to make a baby. Some experts even talk about the "12-month pregnancy," meaning that it's smart to spend at least three months getting yourself ready before you start trying and before you get pregnant. But even if you've already embarked on your babymaking project, it's never too late to take steps to improve your health, and your future child's. Go through the dozen suggestions on this list and check them off one-by-one as you make the changes. Consider it your own countdown to conception. Ready, set, go!

Start taking a daily vitamin containing at least 400 micrograms of folic acid.

Folic acid, also called vitamin B9, is one of the most important supplements a pre-pregnant woman can take. Taking this vitamin before pregnancy can help prevent some devastating birth defects, including spina bifida (in which the developing spinal column doesn't close properly). In fact, it's estimated that if all women of reproductive age took folic acid supplements before getting pregnant and during early pregnancy, as many as 70 percent of these cases could be prevented. Don't wait until you're pregnant to start. The neural tube—the earliest version of the spinal cord—develops very early in pregnancy, before many women even realize they're pregnant.

Pre-Conception Checklist

Schedule a preconception checkup.

Ideally, women should see their doctor three to four months before they conceive. That allows enough time to get vaccines for rubella (German measles) and varicella (chicken pox) if they're needed. But the preconception medical visit is much more than just shots. This is also the time for the doctor to check you out thoroughly so that any potential problems can be anticipated and avoided before pregnancy. For instance, if your doctor knows you've had a sexually transmitted disease in the past, she may decide to check for blockages of the fallopian tubes that might inhibit conception.

Schedule a checkup for your partner, too.

Have your partner visit his physician for a thorough checkup, too. There's probably no need for a sperm test at this point, unless the doctor sees the potential for problems. But making sure that general health is good can help maximize fertility in men and women. In men, for instance, even minor infections with no symptoms can sometimes be enough to affect sperm production. Let a doctor give your partner a clean bill of health before you start trying.

Visit your dentist.

Getting a thorough dental exam before you conceive may be almost as important as your preconception medical checkup. Women with oral and dental problems such as gingivitis (inflammation of the gums) and periodontal disease (more advanced gum disease that can also affect the bone that supports the teeth) are at increased risk of delivering prematurely and having low-birthweight babies. Start brushing and flossing regularly, and see your dentist soon. If you need to have dental work done, you'll want to have any X-rays or other extensive treatments before you conceive.

Get any existing health conditions under control.

Women with thyroid problems, diabetes, hypertension, heart problems, depression, asthma, epilepsy, and other chronic medical conditions can greatly increase their odds of having a healthy pregnancy and baby when their condition is well managed before they conceive. Unchecked hypertension (high blood pressure), for instance, can impair blood flow to a fetus, and untreated asthma can reduce oxygen flow.

Give yourself a medicine makeover.

It's not just women with chronic conditions who may need to review their medications. It's wise to check out any medications you take before embarking on a quest to get pregnant. Take a better-safe-than-sorry attitude and tell your doctor about all the remedies you use, whether for serious illnesses, or just occasional headaches and allergy attacks. Don't forget to mention herbs and alternative therapies, too. You may need to spend a few months switching to different medications and making sure they work properly before you can safely try to conceive.

Find out about your family history.

Biology isn't necessarily destiny, but it's smart to learn about your family's— and especially your mother's—reproductive and health histories to see if there are any potential problems that you can anticipate and avoid. For instance, if your mother went through a very early menopause, it might be a smart move if you didn't wait too long before trying to become a mother yourself. And if there are genetic diseases that run in your or your partner's families, you both can be screened for them before pregnancy, to know whether your baby will be at risk.

Pre-Conception Checklist

Make sure your environment is fertility-friendly.

We live in a chemical world, and some of those chemicals may not be safe or healthy for developing babies (or the eggs and sperm that create them). In particular, scientists have raised concerns about phthalates—a class of chemicals used in cosmetics and plastics—and bisphenol A, another plastics chemical. Take a look at your home and job environment, and see what you can do to reduce your chemical exposures. For instance, you can stop using plastic plates and eating utensils, switch to "green" cleaning products, and look for "natural" cosmetics without harmful ingredients.

Start a fertility diet.

If you want to be a mother, it's time to make sure your diet is fertility-friendly. Good choices include beans and other sources of vegetable protein, whole grains (rather than refined carbs), unsaturated fats (olive oil, peanut oil, canola oil, nuts, fish), and iron-rich fruits and vegetables. Avoid unhealthy trans fats (in hydrogenated oils and many processed foods), soft drinks, and lots of red meat or poultry.

Learn about the weight to be pregnant.

Mothers come in all shapes and sizes, but you've got the best chance of an easy conception and healthy pregnancy if you are at a healthy weight before you conceive. Women who are overweight or obese are at increased risk for pregnancy complications such as diabetes, hypertension, preterm delivery, and cesarean section. And since trying to lose weight while you're pregnant isn't a good idea, it's best to slim down before you conceive. Being underweight isn't fertility-friendly, either. If you're too thin, try to gain a few pounds even before you get that positive pregnancy test.

Kick your bad habits now.

Not only is smoking bad for your baby once you're pregnant, but if you smoke while you're trying, it might take you longer to conceive. And if you wind up needing fertility treatments, smoking can interfere with their success, too. So don't postpone quitting until after the pregnancy test is positive: butt out now! As for drinking, there's no amount of alcohol that's considered safe during pregnancy. For that reason, some doctors think it's smart for women to stop drinking while they're trying.

Last but not least, set a date to ditch the birth control.

If you're using barrier methods of contraception, like the condom, diaphragm, or cervical cap, you can continue using them right up until the day you want to begin trying to conceive. These methods don't have any lasting effects on the body. But if you use hormonal methods of contraception—the Pill, patch, rod, ring, shot, or IUD—you might want to stop a little earlier and substitute a barrier method until you're ready. Studies show that fertility is restored fairly quickly after oral contraceptives are stopped, but it may take longer with other hormonal methods. And many doctors advise women to wait for at least one normal menstrual period/cycle before getting pregnant, since that makes it easier to date the pregnancy and predict the due date.

Pre-Conception Checklist

Resources

This book provides information about general reproductive health, natural conception, and various kinds of fertility treatments, including ART (assisted reproductive technology, which includes in vitro fertilization). For anyone who wants more information than can fit in these pages, there are other resources available.

There are Web sites, organizations, and other books that can provide more information on specific questions, problems, and concerns that you might have. Here are a few good information sources to check out (keep in mind that none of these, of course, is a substitute for medical advice):

ORGANIZATIONS AND WEB SITES

Conceive Magazine

Conceive Magazine and Conceive Online provide information and support for women at any stage of family-building. www.conceiveonline.com

American Academy of Obstetricians and Gynecologists (ACOG)

The Web site of this national organization of women's health care physicians provides patient information on all aspects of reproduction. www.acog.org

The American Fertility Association (AFA)

The AFA, a not-for-profit organization, provides information about infertility treatments, reproductive and sexual health, and family-building options, including surrogacy and adoption. www.theafa.org

American Society for Reproductive Medicine (ASRM)

An organization of specialists in reproductive medicine, the ASRM's Web site provides a wealth of information on infertility and its treatments. www.asrm.org

Centers for Disease Control and Prevention (CDC)

This is a government agency site for a preconception care public health campaign urging women of reproductive age to get themselves healthy before becoming pregnant. A good resource for general and reproductive health information. www.cdc.gov/ncbddd/preconception

Fertile Hope

This nonprofit organization is dedicated to helping cancer patients who are facing infertility after diagnosis and treatment. www.fertilehope.org

Fertility LifeLines

An educational service provided by Serono, a pharmaceutical company. Callers to Fertility LifeLines speak to representatives, including nurse specialists, who can answer questions about fertility health concerns. www.fertilitylifelines.com, 1-866-LETS-TRY

The InterNational Council on Infertility Information Dissemination (INCIID)

INCIID (pronounced "inside") is a nonprofit organization that helps individuals and couples explore their family-building options. INCIID also offers scholarships for families that need help financing treatment. www.inciid.org

March of Dimes

This not-for-profit organization aims to improve the health of babies by educating the public about preconception and prenatal health and how to prevent birth defects, premature birth, and infant mortality. www.marchofdimes.com

RESOLVE: The National Infertility Association

Resolve is a nonprofit organization for men and women experiencing fertility disorders. The group has a network of chapters nationwide to promote reproductive health and raise awareness of infertility issues and family-building options. www.resolve.org

BOOKS

GENERAL REPRODUCTIVE HEALTH AND NATURAL CONCEPTION:

The Fertility Journal: A Day-by-Day Guide to Getting Pregnant

By Kim Hahn and the Editors of *Conceive Magazine* (Chronicle Books, 2008)
A daily fill-in journal full of information about diet, exercise, lifestyle, fertility treatments, and other factors that can influence conception.
www.thefertilityjournal.com

Before Your Pregnancy: A 90-Day Guide for Couples on How to Prepare for a Healthy Conception

By Amy Ogle, MS, RD, and Lisa Mazzullo, MD (Ballantine Books, 2002) Mazzullo, an obstetrician, and Ogle, a dietitian, exercise physiologist, and personal trainer, lead readers through the lifestyle changes to make and medical issues to consider during the three months before conception (or "trying") to give the best odds for a healthy pregnancy.

The Everything Getting Pregnant Book

By Robin Elise Weiss (Adams Media Corporation, 2004) Weiss, a certified childbirth educator, outlines the path to pregnancy, from going off birth control to considering fertility treatments.

Fertility and Conception

By Zita West (DK Adult, 2003) A well-known British midwife (also author of *Plan to Get Pregnant*, DK Adult, 2008) with a holistic approach, West provides advice for couples who are newly trying as well as those who are experiencing problems. The book also discusses fertility treatment options, including IVF, neatly bridging the divide between conventional medicine and alternative treatments.

The Fertility Diet

By Jorge Chavarro, MD, Walter C. Willett, MD, and Patrick J. Skerrett (The McGraw-Hill Companies, Inc., 2008) Research results from the *Nurses' Health Study* at the Harvard School of Public Health indicate diet and lifestyle factors that boost ovulation and improve the chances of getting pregnant.

The Mother of All Pregnancy Books

By Ann Douglas (Wiley, 2002) A remarkably well-researched and comprehensive book that begins with information for couples considering pregnancy and continues all the way through to delivery and breast-feeding.

Preconception Plain and Simple

By Audrey Couto McClelland and Sharon K. Couto (Pinks and Blues Publishing, 2005) A fun book for couples just embarking on the fertility journey, this mother-daughter team of authors provides information on promoting fertility with foods, flowers, aromas, gemstones, and amulets. The idea is to follow the usual medical advice (provided), and then add a bit of romance and relaxation to conception.

Taking Charge of Your Fertility

By Toni Weschler, MPH (Collins, Tenth Anniversary Edition, 2006) This classic fertility tome explains how to use the fertility awareness method (FAM) to achieve or avoid pregnancy. By observing various fertility signs like morning temperature and cervical mucus, women learn to determine when they are ovulating.

FERTILITY CHALLENGES:

Conquering Infertility

By Alice D. Domar, PhD, and Alice Lesch Kelly (Penguin, 2004) Domar, an assistant professor of medicine at Harvard, gives women the tools they need to deal with the stress that can undermine fertility or arise from infertility. Topics include relaxation techniques such as yoga, meditation, journal writing, and guided imagery.

The Fertile Female

By Julia Indichova (Adell Press, 2007) Indichova, also author of *Inconceivable: A Woman's Triumph over Despair and Statistics* (Broadway, 2001), espouses a hopeful and empowering view of female fertility. The book includes nurturing advice as well as information on a fertility-friendly lifestyle and diet (including recipes).

I Am More Than My Infertility

By Marina Lombardo and Linda J. Parker (Seeds of Growth Press, 2007) Lombardo, *Conceive Magazine*'s "Emotionally Speaking" columnist, provides information and psychological support for women dealing with fertility challenges.

The Infertility Answer Book

By Brette McWhorter Sember (Sphinx Publishing, 2005) Sember, an attorney, answers the legal questions surrounding fertility treatments, third-party reproduction (donor egg, donor sperm, surrogates, and gestational carriers), and adoption. Along with medical advice, this book can help couples decide how to proceed when natural conception doesn't work.

The Infertility Cure

By Randine Lewis (Little, Brown and Company, 2005) Lewis is a licensed acupuncturist and herbalist, and her book espouses Chinese medicine as an alternative to conventional Western treatments.

100 Questions & Answers about Infertility

By John D. Gordon, MD, and Michael DiMattina, MD (Jones and Bartlett Publishers, 2007) Two doctors answer the kinds of questions that couples struggling with fertility problems want to know the answers to.

Fertility Facts

Conceptions and Misconceptions

By Arthur L. Wisot, MD, and David R. Meldrum, MD (Hartley and Marks Publishers, revised and expanded second edition, 2004) Two fertility specialists guide readers through the world of high-tech reproductive treatments, including tips for evaluating infertility clinics.

In Vitro Fertilization: The A.R.T. of Making Babies

By Geoffrey Sher, MD, Virginia Marriage Davis, RN, MN, and Jean Stoess, MA (Facts on File, third edition, 2005) A complete guide to IVF, including information for couples on how to determine whether they're eligible for treatment, how to select a good program, and an in-depth guide to how the technology works.

What to Do When You Can't Get Pregnant

By Daniel A. Potter, MD, and Jennifer S. Hanin, MD (Marlow & Company, 2005) This book outlines all the reasons why couples may have trouble conceiving naturally, and then describes the gamut of low- and high-tech methods available to help. There's also a fascinating chapter on future and experimental technologies, such as stem cell research and cloning.

Index

A

abortions, effect on fertility, 18, 90

acne medications (isotretinoins), avoid using, 26

acupuncture, and fertility, 95, 156
  male fertility and, 203

African Americans, sickle cell anemia and, 21

alcohol, cutting consumption of, 137, 206, 297

anemia, 152

angelica (dong quai), 155

anorexia and bulimia, 112

antidepressants, and fertility, 24, 217

antihistamines, and fertility, 24

antihypertensives, and male fertility, 217

assisted reproductive technology (ART), 245-283, 288
  See also IVF (in vitro fertilization)
  success rate using, 265
  using donor eggs, 261, 263

B

basal body temperature (BBT), charting, 61, 237, 285

belly dancing, 166

biological clock, 11, 189

birth control. *See* contraceptives

birth control pills, 32-34
  polycystic ovary syndrome and, 34

births, 75, 77
  average age of women in U.S. giving, 63

black cohosh (herbal remedy), 155

blood thinners (Warfarin), avoid taking, 26

BMI (body mass index), 171
  being overweight and, 173, 262
  male fertility and, 222

body shape, and fertility, 38, 159

books recommended, 301-305

breast cancer, and ovulation disorder, 270

C

caffeine, cutting back intake of, 134-135, 196

Canavan (disease), genetic testing for, 21

cancer survivors, and fertility, 106

carnitine supplements, male fertility and, 198

celiac disease, 111

cell phone use, and fertility, 11, 212

cereal, as source for folic acid, 139

chasteberry (herbal supplement), 145, 156

chemical toxins, and fertility, 91

chicken pox, vaccine to protect against, 19

chronic health conditions, 16, 25

cinnamon, benefits of, 138

clomiphene citrate (medication), 275

coffee drinking, cutting back on, 134, 195

conception. *See also* fertility
  giving it time before seeking treatment, 69
  odds of, 48, 51
  preconception checklist, 293-297
  preconception checkup, 16, 17, 18, 294
  preparing for, 15
  reducing stress to improve chances of, 83

contraceptives, 31-34, 37, 297

corticosteroids, and fertility, 24

cystic fibrosis, genetic testing for, 21

D

dairy products, 11, 132
  may influence chances of having twins, 125
  whole vs. skim milk, 11, 132

dancing, positive impact of, 93

darkness, benefits of, 94
  wearing blue-blocking glasses, 94

decongestants, and fertility, 24

dental health, 28, 294
  bleaching your teeth, 29
  gingivitis, 28
  periodontitis (gum disease), 28

Fertility Facts

Index

recommended rate of intercourse, 231

sperm leakage after sex, 241

sexually transmitted diseases (STDs), 18, 102, 207

chlamydia, 31, 102, 207

contraception reducing the risk of, 31

gonorrhea, 31, 102

smoking, and fertility, 18, 85, 99, 257, 297

male fertility and, 17, 86, 200

why bad for fertility, 85

soft drinks, cutting back consumption of, 135

soy products, avoid consumption of, 11, 123, 190

sperm. See male fertility

stress, and fertility, 17, 22, 82, 83, 223, 278

sunlight, and fertility, 87

surrogate mothers, 264

swimming pool, old wives' tale about, 240

T

Tay-Sachs disease, genetic testing for, 21

teeth. See dental health

testosterone, 70, 107

tetanus/diphtheria vaccinations, 19

thalassemias, alpha and beta, genetic testing and, 21

thyroid conditions and fertility, 25, 104, 105

Traditional Chinese Medicine (TCM), 12, 155, 156, 203

trans fat, and fertility, 126

tubal ligation, reversing, 30

twins, 125, 149

U-V

unsaturated fats, benefits of, 127

urine test for ovulation, 71

uterus, malformed, 113

vacation, taking one to help with conception, 96

vaccinations, being up-to-date on, 19

varicoceles (varicose veins in the scrotum), 226

vasectomy reversals, 218

vegans and vegetarians, 125, 128

Viagra, and male fertility, 202

vitamin A, caution regarding, 150

vitamin B-12, 151

vitamins and supplements, 141-157

herbal supplements, 148, 155

multivitamins, 142-143

prenatal, 23, 142, 157

reading the label, 154

water soluble, 154

W-X-Y-Z

Web sites, list of recommended, 299-301

weight, and fertility, 177, 296

avoiding crash diets, 175

being overweight, 173, 174, 262

being underweight, 172

polycystic ovary syndrome (PCOS) and, 108, 173, 176

women (by decade) and fertility

in their 20s, 52

in their 30s, 53

in their 40s, 40, 49, 54

women over 35, 49, 54

mother's fertility history, 40

quality of eggs, 50

seeing a fertility specialist, 250

sixth month shortcut, 250

test for egg supply, 27, 40, 49

world's oldest mother, 55

workplace environmental hazards, 36, 92, 219

yoga, and fertility, 84, 163, 168

zinc (mineral supplement), 147, 197

Index

Acknowledgments

I'm so very proud that *Conceive*'s message is now expanding into new media. It started with *Conceive Magazine* in 2004, then Conceive On-Air in 2006, and Conceive Online in 2007. *Fertility Facts* is our second book, following *The Fertility Journal: A Day-by-Day Guide to Getting Pregnant* (Chronicle Books, 2008). These books, along with all of Conceive's other media outlets, will help bring the message of health, fertility, and family-building to even more women and couples.

As with all books, many people's work is responsible for what lies between the covers. For this book, first and foremost, we'd like to thank the many writers who have contributed their research and hard work to filling the pages of *Conceive Magazine* with interesting and accurate information to help couples on their journey to parenthood. In addition, special thanks go to Alyson McNutt English, Katherine Johnson, Leslie Laurence, Shari Sims, and Robin Street, who took much of that information and put it into the form you see here. And a big thank you to Lisa Campbell, our editor at Chronicle Books, who has worked with *Conceive*'s staff to help bring the message of the magazine to a new and wider audience.

Finally, I have to acknowledge the hard-working members of the Conceive team who work day in and day out to make these projects a reality. I also want to thank my daughter Taylor, whose journey to me and my husband inspired me to change my career and dedicate myself to all who desire the loving family of their dreams.